W9-AHV-040

Scholarships
and Loans
for
Nursing Education
1997-1998

Pub. No. 41-7300

NLN Press • New York

Copyright 1997 by
National League for Nursing
350 Hudson Street, New York, NY 10014

All rights reserved. No part of this book may be
reproduced in print, or by photostatic means, or in
any other manner, without the express written
permission of the publisher.

ISBN 0-88737-730-0

This book was set in Galliard by
Publications Development Company, Crockett, Texas.
The editor was Regina Fawcett.
Book Crafters was the printer.

Printed in the United States of America

Contents

Goal: Nursing Education or Research

Nursing is an exciting career with many different opportunities for those who have acquired the necessary education and skills. Still, the decision to begin or continue your nursing education, or to advance your standing in the profession through research, is a big one. Figuring out how you will finance your studies or research is part of that decision.

You should not be discouraged from your goals by lack of funds. Although some funds for education or research have been shrinking in recent years, federal and state resources are still available. For students, public sources for financial aid include federal and state scholarships and loans as well as work study programs. Many schools and universities have their own financial aid packages as well. Finally, all sorts of community groups and membership organizations offer their own scholarships and loans for a variety of special purposes and for specific constituencies. For researchers, there are many public and private sources for grants and fellowships as well. This book is designed to help you explore these and other sources of financial aid.

In terms of financing your nursing education, you will be most successful if you start early to apply for aid and put time and effort into your search. Start by choosing the school you wish to attend. The following chapter of this book will talk about your options in nursing education and give you some guidelines for making that choice. Next, we will describe how to apply for financial aid. Most financial aid comes through the schools themselves, which administer

1

federal and state funds as well as school or university scholarships. Most of this aid is awarded to students based on their need for financial assistance, not just on merit. The chapter on the financial aid package will describe the different types of aid for which you may be eligible.

In terms of financing your research endeavors through grants or fellowships, you too should start early in determining the program or institution you wish to proceed with. In the chapter devoted to special awards, postdoctoral study, and research grants you will find important information to help you clarify your options and make your choices.

The bulk of this book is devoted to listings of scholarships, fellowships, grants, traineeships, and loans that are specifically intended for nursing education and research. A numerical code next to the heading for each listing will tell you which groups of nursing students and professionals are eligible to apply for that program. (That code is explained on page 17.) In addition, separate chapters list specific sources of assistance for minority students, and special grants and traineeships for research and postdoctoral study. A final chapter lists the scholarships and loans available from NLN's constituent leagues for nursing. An appendix provides a directory of state boards of nursing. The different indexes at the back of the book make it easy to find all the programs that offer aid for your educational level or for your particular area of interest in nursing.

It's a good idea to read through the entire book, not just the individual listings, to get an understanding of the many ways to finance a nursing education or research endeavor. The Resource section at the end of the book also lists information about other useful publications to help you find all possible sources of assistance. Some of these publications can help you work through the maze of forms that your financial aid applications may require. Others provide comprehensive listings of aid from many specific sources that can be of use to particular groups of applicants, or to institutions of higher education and research through which many grants, fellowships, and traineeships flow. A well-stocked public or school library will have many of these publications. In many cities now as well special Foundation Center or Grant Center libraries have opened for your use. Time spent in researching sources of financial aid and following through with your applications long before you plan to begin your studies or research will be well worthwhile for students whose goal is a career in nursing and for professionals seeking to enhance their career status through research.

Choosing a School

There are many roads to a career in nursing. If you are beginning your nursing education, first learn about the different types of programs available—baccalaureate degree, associate degree, diploma, and practical nursing. To become a registered nurse (RN), you must pass a licensing exam offered by your state board of nursing. A candidate can become eligible to take the exam by graduating from either a two-year associate degree program, a three-year diploma program, or a four-year baccalaureate program approved by the state board of nursing. However, educational preparation often determines salary and mobility within the field of nursing.

The basic baccalaureate program combines nursing courses with general education in a four-year curriculum in a senior college or university. Baccalaureate graduates are able to take positions in community health, progress into administration and advanced nursing, and continue their education at the graduate level. Certain specialties in nursing require a minimum of a baccalaureate degree. Many schools of nursing also offer special programs for nurses who have received their basic nursing education in another type of program and now wish to obtain a bachelor's degree.

Associate degree programs vary in length from two academic years to two calendar years and are offered at public or private community or junior colleges as well as some senior colleges and technical institutes. The program of study combines nursing courses and supportive college courses. Associate degree graduates are qualified to work giving direct care in hospitals and similar institutions in the community.

Diploma programs are generally offered under the auspices of a hospital, frequently in cooperation with an educational institution.

These programs are usually three years in length. Diploma graduates are qualified to work giving direct care in hospitals and similar institutions.

A fourth type of nursing program, leading to a career in practical nursing, is usually one to one-and-a-half years in length and is offered at vocational-technical schools or community colleges. These programs qualify the graduate to take the state board of nursing examination for practical nursing. Those who pass become licensed practical nurses (LPNs); in some states they are known as licensed vocational nurses (LVNs). LPNs are qualified to work in hospitals and similar institutions under the supervision of a registered nurse.

Advanced study, often leading to the master's or doctoral degree, is required for many specialties in nursing, such as nurse-midwife or nurse anesthetist, as well as for those who wish to become nurse practitioners, clinical specialists, and, in many cases, nurse administrators and teachers.

Each type of nursing program differs in requirements for entry, length and cost of the program, and the level of practice for which it prepares its graduates. You should investigate the different types of programs thoroughly and decide which one is right for your needs and goals before you apply. NLN Press publications *Nursing: The Career of a Lifetime,* by Shirley Fondiller and B. J. Nerone, and *Managing Your Career in Nursing,* by Francis C. Henderson and Barbara McGettizan, offer much needed information on career choices and the profession of nursing in general. These books will help you make an informed choice. NLN Press also publishes directories of different nursing programs (see Resources section). These publications will help you in finding a program appropriate to your needs.

Once you have decided which type of program suits you best, the next step is to select a particular school. It's a good idea to select several nursing programs that interest you and not to limit your choice to just one school. Faculty and instruction are unique to each school. Laboratory and clinical facilities, cost, location—any number of factors may influence your decision.

Many nurses today are deciding to go back to school to get baccalaureate degrees or to advance their careers through graduate education. Some beginning nursing students are entering nursing school some years after graduating from high school. These students may have work or family obligations that make such considerations important. Some of the publications in the Resources section will be useful for this group as well.

When you have narrowed down your selection, write to the schools of your choice, asking for a catalog, an application form, and information on financial assistance. Keep in mind that applications are usually due at a school in January or February for classes beginning the following September.

Applying for Financial Aid

Most schools today require students who want financial aid (including loans) to complete a need-analysis form, which is a means of estimating a student's need for financial assistance to meet educational expenses. The analysis determines how much money you or your family can contribute to your total educational expenses. The smaller your income, the smaller your individual contribution. Financial aid, as determined by this method, is based solely on need, and not at all on merit. An excellent description of need analysis, including advice for those who don't automatically qualify for need-based assistance, is given in *Don't Miss Out* (see Resources section).

The schools to which you will apply will send you a need-analysis form to fill out even before you are notified of acceptance. Many schools require the same form, so you may need to fill it out only once. Be sure to read all forms thoroughly, because they are complicated. If you make any errors or leave out any information, the form will be returned to you for corrections, so be sure to answer each question completely and accurately. You should fill out the forms as soon as you and your family have collected your financial records for the current tax year. For fall admission, the form should be filed as early as possible after January 1, as soon as the necessary information is complete. Getting this form in early is vital, because the amount of aid available at each school is limited. Schools use the need-analysis report for determining all need-based financial aid.

You will send the completed form to the agency identified on the form which will perform the analysis. Students in basic nursing programs will check the box requesting that one copy be sent to the Department of Education for the Pell Grant. This is the largest of the federal aid programs and is designed for undergraduate students only. You may also check a box to forward the analysis to your state's educational grant office. For a fee, you can have copies of the analysis sent to each of the schools to which you have applied for admission. About six weeks after you have sent in the form for analysis, you will receive a Student Aid Report, which will include an estimate of what you and your family can pay toward your college costs.

Once the amount of your family or personal contribution toward your education is computed by the need analysis, it will remain the same, regardless of which schools you apply to or what their tuition and fees are. For example, the need analysis may determine that your income will allow you to pay $2,000 a year toward your educational costs. In this case, your family or individual contribution will always be $2,000, whether the school you wish to attend has annual tuition and fees of $4,000 or $20,000.

What will vary is your remaining need and the financial assistance that different schools offer you, depending on their resources, the number of applicants, and how early your application is received. The variation in these "financial aid packages," as they are called, is one reason for applying to several schools.

The Financial Aid Package

A school will compute a financial aid package for you only after you have been accepted for admission. Being admitted to a school does not commit you to attend. You can make up your mind after you have compared the assistance that the different schools offer you.

The school's financial aid office will try to make up the difference between your family or individual contribution (as determined by the need analysis) and the cost of the nursing program for a year. The financial aid package will be drawn from federal and state sources available to the school and from the school's own resources. It will usually include grants, loans, and work-study. Most students in need of financial aid accept educational loans (for example, a Perkins Loan—formerly the National Direct Student Loan—charges only 5 percent interest). In fact, according to the College Board, loans now make up half of all financial assistance given to students. In 1994–1995, nearly 50 percent of student aid was in the form of grants, and less than 5 percent was work-study.

FEDERAL SOURCES OF FINANCIAL AID

All federal sources of educational assistance depend on congressional appropriations. The information given here is applicable for the 1997–1998 academic year, and was taken mainly from the free Department of Education brochure, *The Student Guide: Financial Aid from the U.S. Department of Education 1997–1998* (see Resources section). Students who are planning several years of study should not count on having all the financial assistance described here in future years. NLN-accredited nursing programs are eligible to participate in all of the federal aid programs. For eligibility of other programs, consult school catalogs or financial aid offices.

THE PELL GRANT

Beginning Study Only. This is the major federal program for education, and it assists students who demonstrate need for financial assistance to study in any type of basic nursing program or other fields of undergraduate study. Grants for 1997–1998 range up to $2,470 a year. The size of your award will depend on your need for assistance, the cost of tuition and fees at your school, and other factors. The amount calculated for your Pell Grant will be applied to your financial aid package by any school eligible to participate in the Pell Grant program (financial aid officers or the school catalog will tell you whether a school is eligible to participate). You must complete the need-analysis form to determine your eligibility. Students may apply for Pell awards for each year of study, but the program depends on congressional appropriations. These grants need not be repaid. Students may request a free copy of *The Student Guide: Financial Aid From the U.S. Department of Education 1996–1997* from the U.S. Department of Education. Applications and general student financial assistance information may be requested from the Federal Student Aid Information Center, P.O. Box 84, Washington, DC 20044. Telephone (800) 4-FED AID. Apply for Pell Grants as soon as possible after January 1. Student aid applications must be received by the appropriate processor no later than May 1.

SUPPLEMENTAL EDUCATIONAL OPPORTUNITY GRANTS (SEOG)

Beginning Study Only. Students must be enrolled at least half-time as regular students in an eligible undergraduate program of study at a school that participates in the SEOG program. They must be U.S. citizens or eligible noncitizens. Only students of exceptional financial need are eligible for these grants, which award up to

$4,000 for a year's study in a basic nursing program (or any other undergraduate program) and require no payback. The amount is determined by schools eligible to participate in the program. Participating schools have a set amount of SEOG funds to distribute among students with demonstrated need; thus, it is important to apply early.

COLLEGE WORK-STUDY PROGRAM

Beginning Study and RNs. Another program supported by the federal government provides funds for part-time employment, on or off campus, in colleges and universities participating in the program. Students work at a salary at least equal to the current minimum wage, and always for public or nonprofit organizations. The school arranges a job and sets the number of hours to be worked. Awards are made by the financial aid office on the basis of demonstrated need. Submit completed applications to postsecondary educational institutions early in the calendar year.

NURSING STUDENT LOAN PROGRAM
U.S. DEPARTMENT OF HEALTH AND HUMAN SERVICES

Beginning Study and RNs. For nursing students in particular, loans of up to $2,500 per academic year (freshmen and sophomores) and up to $4,000 (juniors and seniors), based on financial need, are available for basic or graduate study in participating schools of nursing. Repayment of these low-interest loans begins nine months after a student graduates or leaves school. Students are allowed up to ten years to repay the loan, and during the repayment period they will be charged 5 percent interest (for all loans made on or after November 4, 1988). Students apply to their school of nursing, and loan recipients are selected by the participating schools.

PERKINS LOANS (formerly NATIONAL DIRECT STUDENT LOANS)

Beginning Study, RNs, and Graduate Study. Participating schools act as the lenders for these loans, which are funded by the federal government. Students in most nursing programs who demonstrate need and are attending school at least half-time are eligible for them. (One-year practical nursing programs are not eligible to participate.) Students may borrow up to $3,000 for the first two years of study and up to $9,000 after two years of study in a baccalaureate program, minus what was borrowed for the first two years of study. If you choose to go on to graduate study, you may borrow up to $15,000, minus the total of what you borrowed for undergraduate study. Repayment begins nine months after a student graduates or leaves school for new borrowers or after six months for continuing borrowers, at a 5 percent interest rate. The loan may be repaid over a period of ten years, but under certain circumstances, repayment may be deferred.

STAFFORD LOANS (formerly GUARANTEED STUDENT LOANS)/PLUS LOANS/SLS LOANS

Beginning Study, RNs, and Graduate Study.   Another program backed by state guarantee agencies or the federal government makes loans available to students who are new borrowers at 8 percent interest. Students must arrange these loans privately through banks, credit unions, savings and loan associations, or other commercial lenders. (The federal government's publication, *The Student Guide,* lists guarantee agencies in each state, with addresses and telephone numbers, to inform you about this loan program.)

Under the Stafford Loan program, students in basic education programs may borrow as much as $2,625 a year in the first and second years and $3,500–$5,500 a year after that, with a limit of $23,000 for the entire period of study. Graduate students may borrow up to $8,500 a year for a total of $65,000, including loans for undergraduate study. Students must demonstrate financial need to be eligible for the Stafford Loan.

Repayment usually begins six months after the student graduates or leaves school, and borrowers have a liberal amount of time in which to repay the loan. Under certain circumstances, repayment may be deferred or canceled. Student borrowers are charged a 5 percent loan-origination fee, which is deducted from the amount received. The lending institution may also charge an additional insurance premium of up to 3 percent of the loan principal.

Under the PLUS (for parents of dependent children) and SLS (for independent students) loan programs, amounts of educational loans of up to $4,000 per year for a total of $23,000 at a maximum interest rate of 3 percent of the loan principal are available. No loan origination fee is charged, and PLUS and SLS are not based on individual need. However, while PLUS borrowers do not have to show need, they may have to undergo a credit analysis. SLS, on the other hand, is based on eligibility requirements that are available at the financial aid office of your institution of choice. Repayment begins 60 days after the loan goes into effect.

SUPPLEMENTAL LOANS FOR STUDENTS (formerly ALAS)

Beginning Study, RNs, and Graduate Study. Graduate and independent undergraduate students are eligible for loans of up to $4,000 per year, for a maximum of $20,000, in addition to Stafford Loan funds. Loans are not need-based, but the total amount borrowed in any year cannot be greater than the cost of education minus all other aid received. The annual interest rate is set by a formula tied to the rate of the 52-week U.S. Treasury bill plus 3.25 percent, not to exceed 12 percent. Interest payments must be made quarterly while you are in school, and repayment of principal begins when you are no longer enrolled full-time.

STATE SOURCES OF FINANCIAL AID

All states have need-based grants for education, and some of them allow grants for study outside the state. Most of the need-based aid will be administered by the school, and the financial aid office will include this source in making up your financial aid package.

For example, the New York State Higher Education Services Corporation (99 Washington Avenue, Albany, NY 12255) provides **Tuition Assistance Program (TAP)** grants for New York State residents in full-time degree-granting programs. The awards are based on need and range from $350 to $4,125 per year for dependent undergraduates and $100 to $1,200 per year for dependent graduate students. TAP awards are also available for independent graduate and undergraduate students. Various **New York State Opportunity Program** grants are available to academically and economically disadvantaged state residents attending New York State institutions. Applications for these programs are usually distributed to high school seniors or made through the college financial aid office.

In addition, the New York State Department of Health (Corning Tower, Room 1602, Empire State Plaza, Albany, NY 12237) is offering **New York State Health Service Corps Scholarships** of up to $15,000 per year for one or two years of study for students, including those studying to be registered nurses, who are willing to commit themselves to 18 months of service as a health care professional in exchange for each year of funding. Scholarship recipients will become part of a State Health Service Corps to provide service in areas and facilities where there are shortages of personnel, such as state-operated facilities for the mentally ill or prison populations.

New York State also administers a variety of other programs for Native Americans, Vietnam veterans, children of veterans, police officers and firefighters, and other groups.

State programs can be an important source of assistance for nursing students. Each state has a different financial aid program. You can learn about your state's program by writing the appropriate education agency in your state. Your city, town, or community may have financial aid information as well. The local chamber of commerce is a good place to start to find out.

OTHER SOURCES OF FINANCIAL AID

Many schools have need-based funds to assist students, as well as merit-based scholarships. This is more common for private schools than for public ones, but even public schools are establishing alumni funds to provide loans and scholarships for students in need of financial assistance. The financial aid office or the school catalog will inform you about whether a school has its own sources of need-based aid.

Some sources are eligible for **United Student Aid Funds**. This private, not-for-profit corporation guarantees loans made to students by commercial lenders when students are unable to get loans from other sources. Telephone (800) 824-7044.

   In addition to the sources of aid specifically designed for nursing students, which will be detailed in the following chapters, there are many private sources of aid that help particular groups of individuals—for example, minority groups or women. All sorts of organizations sponsor scholarships: employers, unions, fraternal groups, religious and ethnic groups, community organizations, veterans groups—the list could go on and on. Be resourceful! Contact every organization that you and your family are involved with. Some of the publications listed in the Resources section will help you in this search. Ask your high school counselor and the financial aid officer at your new school for help. A little research can pay off in helping to make your nursing education goal a reality.

Scholarships and Loans for Nursing Education

The sources of financial aid for nursing education that are listed in this chapter are many and varied. Some are open to applications from any nursing student; others are designed for study in a particular nursing specialty or at a specific level of nursing education; others still are broader in scope and designed for study in health care professions that include nursing.

The programs that offer scholarships or loans are listed alphabetically. The numerical codes next to each heading will help you determine whether the aid the organization offers is appropriate for your needs. The following categories are used to indicate which groups of nursing students are eligible to apply:

1. Beginning RN study
2. LPN study
3. Baccalaureate completion for RNs
4. Advanced clinical study for RNs
5. Graduate study (master's or doctoral)
6. Doctoral study only
7. Special grants, research, traineeships, or postdoctoral work
8. For minority students primarily

You can consult the indexes to find listings of all the programs in each category. The indexes will also give you a quick rundown of all the programs listed in the chapters on aid for minority students, aid for postdoctoral students, and those interested in doing research or special projects, and aid from NLN's constituent leagues for nursing. If you are interested in a particular specialty or area in nursing, be sure to check the Nursing Specialties index. You can't always tell from the name of an organization what its area of emphasis is.

The time and effort you put into applying to the appropriate sources listed in this book can pay off by reducing your individual contribution to your educational costs, although it may not always do so. Some scholarships go directly to the student. Some schools match the amount of the scholarship with their own funds. Other schools are short of funds for student aid, and the extra scholarship or grant you can obtain on your own may make it possible for you to attend a school with a program of studies that particularly suits your interests and goals. It is possible, however, that a school may include the amount of your scholarship in the school's contribution, so that the amount you have to pay remains the same. All the same, it is worth your while to read through this chapter carefully, because there are many opportunities here to help nursing students obtain their goals.

We have attempted to identify as many of the available scholarships and loans for nursing education as possible. However, new ones are announced regularly in *N&HC: Perspectives on Community,* the *American Journal of Nursing,* and other nursing journals, which you may find in the library of a nursing program.

The schools themselves may have private scholarships and loans specifically for nursing. As noted in the previous section, some states have merit-based scholarships just for nursing education. When you write to your state education department for information on all of its financial aid programs, include a request for information on nursing education grants.

Some state boards of nursing offer aid to nurses who will practice in that state after completing their education. In addition to the national awards listed here, local chapters of membership and specialty organizations may offer scholarships to members or other nurses who are pursuing studies in line with that organization's goals. Again, it is worth the time to investigate all of these possibilities. Some of the publications listed in the Resources section can help in identifying these local sources of aid.

Hospitals are another source of financial assistance for registered nurses. Many of them offer tuition reimbursement, low-cost loans, and other forms of financial aid to their staff. This book cannot begin to list the hospitals that offer assistance for education or the variety of plans that are offered, but if you are employed at a hospital, you should be certain to ask your employer about tuition-assistance plans. Often, financial assistance from a hospital is conditional upon a service obligation. A few hospitals guarantee payment of full tuition and fees *after* a registered nurse completes an advanced degree—certainly a good plan for RNs while education loans are available at low interest rates to finance an education initially.

AIR FORCE ROTC NURSING SCHOLARSHIPS 1, 3, 5, 8

The Air Force nursing scholarship program helps you pursue a nursing degree to earn an Air Force commission through Air Force ROTC. Nursing scholarships are offered for 1 to 4 years. Only high school seniors or graduates who have not attended college full-time may qualify for the 4-year nursing scholarship. Students in college may apply for the 1- to 3-year scholarship. The Type I scholarships pay full college tuition, most mandatory fees, plus a textbook allowance. The Type II scholarships pay the same benefits except tuition is capped at $9,000 per year. All Air Force ROTC cadets on scholarship receive a $150 monthly nontaxable allowance during the school year. After you have completed all AFROTC program requirements and your degree requirements, you will be commissioned a second lieutenant in the Air Force Nurse Corps and serve 4 years on active duty. Newly commissioned nurses will complete licensing requirements after graduation. For more details, contact an Air Force ROTC unit or write: HQ AFROTC Scholarship Actions Section, 551 E. Maxwell Blvd., Maxwell AFB, AL 36112-6106.

ALPHA TAU DELTA   1, 2, 3, 4, 5, 6
NATIONAL FRATERNITY FOR
PROFESSIONAL NURSES

Graduate and undergraduate students who are members in good standing of a university or college chapter of Alpha Tau Delta may apply for grants. All applicants must show evidence of need and submit professional recommendations. Undergraduate applicants must have a grade point average of 2.5 or better. Criteria for awards include degree of financial need, interest in and support of the fraternity, other professional activities, and academic record. Applications must be received on or before April 15, and announcement of recipients will be made by August 1. Further information and applications are available from: National Vice President, National Awards Committee Chairperson, Alpha Tau Delta, 5207 Mesada Street, Alta Loma, CA 91737. Telephone (909) 980-3536.

AMERICAN ASSOCIATION OF CRITICAL CARE 3, 5, 6, 8 NURSES (AACN) SCHOLARSHIPS FOR GRADUATE STUDY IN CARDIOVASCULAR NURSING

Through the support of Kontron Instruments, the AACN will award a scholarship in the spring for graduate study in cardiovascular nursing.

Eligibility requirements for a **Kontron-AACN Cardiovascular Scholarship** are as follows: current RN licensure and graduation from an NLN-accredited bachelors degree program with a nursing major; proof of admission or enrollment in a planned master's or doctoral program with a concentration in cardiovascular nursing; a B average (GPA of 3.0 or higher on a 4.0 scale) or its equivalent in a previous degree or in a current program; current AACN membership; currently working in a critical care unit or worked in one for at least one of the past three years (primary patient and family population should be those with cardiovascular problems); and agree to participate in a follow-up study of the impact of your graduate degree on the care of patients and families in cardiovascular critical care units.

The scholarship can be used for tuition, fees, books, or supplies. Applications must be received by May 15th. For more information and an application, write the AACN National Office, 101 Columbia, Aliso Viejo, CA 92656-1491. Telephone (714) 362-2000, ext. 376.

AMERICAN ASSOCIATION OF NURSE   4, 5 ANESTHETISTS

AANA makes loans of up to $2,500 to student nurse anesthetists who encounter unexpected expenses or financial problems. Candidates must have completed twelve months of a program approved by the

For key to codes showing categories of aid, see page 17.

Council on Accreditation of Nurse Anesthesia Education Programs, and must be associate members of AANA. Repayment begins six months after graduation at a rate of $125 per month, plus 7 percent interest on the unpaid balance. Interest begins to accrue one month after graduation. Send inquiries to: Finance Director, American Association of Nurse Anesthetists, 222 S. Prospect Avenue, Park Ridge, IL 60068-5790.

AMERICAN ASSOCIATION OF OCCUPATIONAL HEALTH NURSES, INC. (AAOHN)　　3, 4, 7

AAOHN sponsors three annual research awards in the area of occupational health nursing practice and one annual academic scholarship (open only to AAOHN members). The **Mary Louise Brown Research Award** provides $3,000 to an experienced researcher; the **Otis Clap Award** in the amount of $2,000 and the **American Board of Occupational Health Nursing Award** in the amount of $1,000 are open to nursing students and clinical practitioners respectively who are contributing to the occupational health nursing knowledge base. The **Charles J. Turcotte Academic Scholarship** in the amount of $2,000 is open only to AAOHN members currently enrolled in baccalaureate, masters, or doctoral nursing programs. To obtain more information on these AAOHN awards, write to: AAOHN Awards, AAOHN, 50 Lenox Pointe, Atlanta, GA 30324-3176. Telephone (404) 262-1162.

AMERICAN CANCER SOCIETY　　　　　　　　　4, 5, 7

Master's degree students who are studying to teach cancer nursing or to become a clinical specialist in cancer nursing are eligible for American Cancer Society **Scholarships in Cancer Nursing,** which offer $8,000 a year for tuition and subsistence and may be renewed for a second year upon application. Candidates must be enrolled in or applying to an NLN-accredited master's program offering specific educational experience in oncology nursing. A current license to practice as a registered nurse and U.S. citizenship or proof of permanent residence are requirements. At the end of each scholarship year, reports must be submitted by the nurse participant and by the faculty member responsible for the oncology component.

Doctoral students who are preparing to be educators, clinical experts, administrators, and/or researchers in cancer nursing are eligible for awards of $8,000 a year for up to four years. Applicants must be enrolled in or applying for a doctoral degree program in nursing science or a science relevant to nursing. A current license to practice as a registered nurse and U.S. citizenship or proof of permanent residence are requirements. Applicants must project a program of study that integrates oncology nursing and provide evidence of faculty support for the program of study. Applicants must also demonstrate a commitment to cancer nursing as evidenced by recent experience, education, and/or research in the specialty area. At the end of each scholarship year, reports must be submitted by the nurse recipient and the faculty sponsor. Funding for years two through four will be based on evidence of progress in the graduate program described in these reports.

The **Professorship in Oncology Nursing Program** is designed to strengthen the cancer curriculum in graduate and undergraduate education, so as to enhance cancer patient and family care. Awards are made to faculty members for three to five years of curriculum enhancement, and with a maximum award amount per year of $35,000. Full-time faculty with assistant, associate, or full professor rank holding a DSN or equivalent are eligible. For more information, contact: Ginger Krawiec, Director, Clinical Awards, Department of Detection and Treatment, (404) 329-5734. Or write to: professorship in Oncology Nursing, American Cancer Society, 1599 Clifton Rd., NE, Atlanta, GA 30329-4251.

Applications for both programs are due by October 1 for the academic year beginning the following September 1. Forms for application may be obtained from local Institutional Grant offices or from: American Cancer Society, Extramural Grant Department, 1599 Clifton Road, NE, Atlanta, GA 30329-4251. Telephone (404) 329-7558, fax (404) 321-4669, WWW http:// www.cancer.org, e-mail grants@cancer.org.

For key to codes showing categories of aid, see page 17.

AMERICAN HOLISTIC NURSES' ASSOCIATION

1, 3, 4, 5

The **Charlotte McGuire Scholarship Programs** offers two annual academic scholarships to member nurses pursuing graduate and undergraduate nursing education. Applicants must meet minimum membership requirements, submit an application consisting of background information, financial statement, statement of goals for education, and demonstrate an interest in or experience in holistic nursing. Also required are professional and academic references. Applications are accepted between January 1 and March 15 of each year. The scholarships are awarded at the Annual Conference in June. For more information, contact the Charlotte McGuire Scholarship Program, American Holistic Nurses' Association, 4101 Lake Boone Trail, Suite 201, Raleigh, NC 27607. Telephone (800) 278-AHNA.

AMERICAN LEGION

3, 4, 5

Awards from the **Eight and Forty Lung and Respiratory Nursing Scholarships Fund** are made in amounts of $2,500 each to assist registered nurses to secure advanced preparation for positions in supervision, administration, or teaching. Students must have prospects of employment in a specific position with a full-time, direct relationship to lung and respiratory disease prevention and treatment upon completion of their study. Application deadline is May 15 of the calendar year in which the school year begins. Announcements of awards are made by July 1 of the same year. For more information and application, write to: The American Legion Education Program, Box 1055, Indianapolis, IN 46206, Attn: Eight and Forty Scholarships.

The American Legion also offers educational assistance in the form of scholarships designed specifically to enter into or enhance current nursing education in Arizona, Arkansas, California, Georgia, Idaho, Illinois, Iowa, Kansas, Michigan, Minnesota, Nebraska, Nevada, New Hampshire, New Jersey, New York, Ohio, Oregon, South Dakota, Texas, Washington, Wisconsin, and Wyoming. For further information on these and other, more general educational assistance programs, contact The American Legion.

AMERICAN NEPHROLOGY NURSES'   3, 4, 5, 7
ASSOCIATION

The American Nephrology Nurses' Association (ANNA) offers scholarships and fellowships in support of individuals in pursuit of baccalaureate and advanced degrees in nursing and dedicated to contributing to the renal community. For information on specific scholarships and awards, write to: American Nephrology Nurses' Association National Office, East Holly Avenue, Pitman, NJ 08071-0056. Telephone (609) 256-2320.

ARMY ROTC   1, 3

Army ROTC offers four, three, and two-year scholarships on a competitive basis to students pursuing a baccalaureate degree at an NLN accredited school of nursing. Scholarships pay most tuition cost, required educational fees, a flat fee for books, supplies and equipment, and provide a subsistence allowance of up to $1,500 each year the scholarship is in effect. For more information concerning Army ROTC Nursing scholarship opportunities write to: Army ROTC, Nursing Opportunities, Gold QUEST Center, P.O. Box 3279, Warminster, PA 18974-0128 or Chief Nurse, U.S. Army Cadet Command, ATTN: ATCC-N, Fort Monroe, VA 23651. Telephone (800) USA-ROTC.

ASSOCIATION OF OPERATING ROOM NURSES   3, 5, 7

Associate or active RN members of AORN who have maintained their membership for at least one year immediately prior to the application deadline are eligible to apply for a number of scholarships through the association. Candidates pursuing baccalaureate or graduate degrees in nursing must be enrolled in an NLN-accredited program and are required to supply evidence of current enrollment or acceptance in the program. Scholarships provide funds for tuition and registration fees and are awarded on the basis of scholastic merit. Financial need is not a criterion for selection. There are two application periods each year, with a deadline date of May 1 and October 1.

You must be a member of AORN to receive an application. To receive criteria and an application, write to: AORN Scholarship Board, AORN Inc., 2170 So. Parker Road #300, Denver, CO 80231-5711. Telephone (303) 755-6300.

ASSOCIATION OF WOMEN'S HEALTH, OBSTETRIC, AND NEONATAL NURSES

3, 4, 5

AWHONN awards research grants yearly. Research grants are available for up to $3,500, and a research utilization grant is awarded for up to $5,000. Applicants must be AWHONN members at the time of the awarding. The applications must be postmarked by November 1. Interested persons may contact the Research Dept. for current guidelines and an application. For more information, contact: AWHONN, 700 14th Street, NW, Suite 600, Washington, DC, 20005-2019. Telephone (202) 662-1613 or fax-on-demand service (800) 395-7373 items 606, 607, and 608.

BUSINESS AND PROFESSIONAL WOMEN'S FOUNDATION

1, 2, 3

The **New York Life Foundation Scholarship Program for Women in the Health Professions** was established in 1984 to assist women seeking the education necessary for entry or re-entry into the work force or advancement within a career in the field of health care. The Scholarship Program is administered through the Business and Professional Women's Foundation Scholarship Program, which the New York Life Foundation has supported since 1978. The program reflects our desire to help meet the increasing need for trained professionals in the health-care field. Scholarships ranging from $500–$1,000 are awarded for full-time or part-time programs of study.

The applicant must be a woman 25 years of age or older and a citizen of the United States; be officially accepted into an program or course of study at a United States institution; ating within 12 to 24 months from September 1; demon cal need for financial assistance; be studying in one of the

For key to codes showing categories of a

fields; and have a definite plan to use the desired training to upgrade skills for career advancement, to train for a new career field, or to enter or re-enter the job market.

This scholarship program does not cover study at the graduate or doctorate levels, correspondence courses, or non-degreed programs. Officers of the New York Life Insurance Company and members of their immediate families are not eligible to participate in this program.

Applications are available between October 1 and April 1. Application packets must be postmarked on or before April 15. In order to receive more information, submit a business-size, self-addressed, double-stamped envelope to: Scholarships, BPW Foundation, 2012 Massachusetts Avenue, NW, Washington, DC 20036.

COMMISSIONED OFFICER STUDENT TRAINING　　3
AND EXTERN PROGRAM PUBLIC HEALTH
SERVICE U.S. DEPARTMENT OF HEALTH
AND HUMAN SERVICES

The **Public Health Service Commissioned Corps** is a United States uniformed service of professionals in health-related fields. Through its Senior Commissioned Officer Student Training and Extern programs (COSTEP), nursing has been prioritized as a principal focus. COSTEP offers a competitive program designed to financially assist students in BSN or MSN programs during their final year of nursing school in return for an agreement to work for the Public Health Service after graduation. Note that COSTEP does not offer scholarships or grants. Basic aspects of the program include financial assistance, additional support, and minimal payback.

In terms of financial assistance: As an active duty Public Health Service Officer during the senior year, the student receives pay and allowances as an O-1 (Ensign) of approximately $1,900 per month. In terms of additional support: Tuition and fees may also be paid depending on the program (see Indian Health Service programs). In terms of minimal payback: Following graduation the student agrees to work for the Public Health Service for twice the time supported (i.e., an 18-month employment commitment for 9 months financial support).

ᐅ codes showing categories of aid, see page 17.

Assignments upon graduation would be in the Public Health Service programs that supported the student in training. For example, assignments could be in one of the following: an Indian Health Service health center, a Native Hawaiian health center, a public hospital, a migrant health center, a community health center, or a rural health center. Assignees would continue as Commissioned Officers (if qualified) and upon graduation be promoted to the rank of O-2 (Lieutenant Junior Grade) with monthly pay and allowances of over $2,150 plus benefits.

Students may apply no later than April preceding their final year of academic study. For application forms, write to: SR COSTEP, U.S. Public Health Service Recruitment, 8201 Greensboro Drive, Suite 600, McLean, VA 22102. Telephone (800) 279-1605.

THE COMMONWEALTH FUND HEALTHY STEPS FOR YOUNG CHILDREN PROGRAM GRANTS

7

The fund places a priority on the healthy growth of young children, developing the capacities of young people, and improving availability of and access to health care services. This program emphasizes the care of children from birth to age three. The program aims to create new approaches to children's health through the expansion of services for healthcare providers and parents beyond the child's physical care. Local initiatives will involve partnerships including the local funder, a healthcare provider, and the Healthy Steps program. The partnerships will create advice lines, support groups, and educational materials for parents as well as provide children with in-home nurse visits, periodic developmental assessments, and referrals to community resources. The fund's board meets in April, July, and November. Applicants should submit a letter proposing their project and include the amount requested, a description of the problem to be addressed, a proposed schedule and workplan, expected outcomes, and qualifications of people involved. For further information contact: Adrienne Fisher, Director of Grants Management, The Commonwealth Fund, Harkness House, One E. 75th Street, New York, NY 10021-2692. Telephone (212) 535-0400, fax (212) 606-3500, e-mail cmwf@cmwf.org, WWW http://www.cmwf.org.

For key to codes showing categories of aid, see page 17.

DEPARTMENT OF DEFENSE   3, 5
UNITED STATES NAVY

Four financial incentive programs have been authorized by the Department of Defense to assist the Navy in the recruitment and retention of qualified nurses: **Nurse Candidate Program, Nurse Accession Bonus Program, Incentive Special Pay for Certified Registered Nurse Anesthetists (CRNAs), and Naval Reserve Officers Training Corps Scholarship Program.**

The **Nurse Candidate Program** is designed for full-time students enrolled in a baccalaureate degree program. An accession bonus of $5,000 and $500 per month for each month enrolled as a full-time student for a maximum of 24 months is offered. The active duty service obligation for candidates enrolling in the program during the fourth year of nursing school is four years. For candidates enrolling in the program for two years, there is a five-year active duty commitment.

The **Nurse Accession Bonus Program** is for qualified nurses and provides a payment of $5,000 at time of appointment in return for a four-year active duty service agreement. This bonus is in addition to other pay and allowances received by Navy Nurse Corps officers.

The **Incentive Pay for Certified Nurse Anesthetists** offers $15,000 per year for each year of obligated service for all qualified CRNAs.

The **Naval Reserve Offices Training Corps (NROTC) Scholarship Program** offers allowances for tuition, texts, uniforms, and fees in addition to a subsistence stipend of $100 per month for a period not to exceed 40 academic months. The active duty service obligation is for a four year period in addition to four years in a reserve status.

For more information on these and other programs, contact the medical programs officer at a Navy Recruiting District near your home or school or call (800) 327-6289.

DEPARTMENT OF VETERANS AFFAIRS   1, 3, 5, 7
HEALTH PROFESSIONAL SCHOLARSHIP PROGRAM

The Health Professional Scholarship Program offers awards to students enrolled full-time or accepted for enrollment in an NLN-accredited nursing program. Awards will be given to students in the final year of associate degree in nursing; third and fourth year of baccalaureate and entry-level master's degree in nursing; and advanced master's degree students with specialties in gerontology, medical/surgical ambulatory care, adult psychiatric/mental health, rehabilitation, and nursing service administration.

Benefits include funds for tuition and fees, other educational expenses, and a monthly stipend of $767. In return, the participant agrees to be employed as a full-time licensed professional in a VA medical center for a two-year service obligation for benefits received.

Applications for the 1997–1998 school year may be obtained from the Health Professional Scholarship Program, by calling (800) 827-1191 between the dates of March 1 and May 19. Requests received before March 1, or after May 19, cannot be processed. The deadline for accepting applications is the last Tuesday in May. Applicants are notified of their selection status the first week of August.

For more information, contact: Health Professional Scholarship Program. Telephone (800) 827-1191.

FOUNDATION OF THE NATIONAL STUDENT NURSES' ASSOCIATION

1, 3, 8

Breakthrough to Nursing Scholarships are offered annually to ethnic/minority students of color for basic nursing education. In making awards, extra credit goes to members of the National Student Nurses' Association, but all eligible students should apply. Eligibility includes students currently enrolled in state-approved schools of nursing or pre-nursing in associate degree, baccalaureate, general doctorate, and generic master's programs. Applications are available until January 15. Deadline for applications is February 1. For information and applications, send a self-addressed business-size envelope with postage to: Foundation of the National Student Nurses' Association, 555 West 57th Street, New York, NY 10019.

HEALTH CANADA'S NATIONAL HEALTH   5, 6
RESEARCH AND DEVELOPMENT PROGRAM
(NHRDP) PERSONNEL AWARDS (MASTERS,
DOCTORATE, POSTDOCTORATE AND
SCHOLAR LEVELS)

The NHRDP offers personnel awards at the masters, doctoral, post-doctoral and scholar levels to individuals whose research training falls under one of Health Canada's four core business lines (please see NHRDP Personnel Awards Update, November 1996 for further information) and where research results have the potential to impact on policy development, strategic planning, and/or program management. All applications must be submitted by March 1, 5:00 PM, EST. For more information, contact: Information Resource Officer, Research and Program Policy Directorate, Health Promotion and Programs Branch, Jeanne Mance Building, Tunney's Pasture, Ottawa, Ontario, K1A 1B4, Canada. Telephone (613) 954-8549, fax (613) 954-7363, e-mail nhrdpinfo@isdtcp3.hwc.ca. The internet address is http://www.hwc.ca/datahpsb/nhrdp.

JAMES S. KEMPER FOUNDATION   1, 3, 5

Kemper Foundation nursing scholarships are available at only four schools of nursing and are administered directly through these schools, which also handle the selection process. Applicants must be enrolled in one of the following schools: Baylor University School of Nursing, Dallas, TX; Crouse-Irving Memorial Hospital, Syracuse, NY; Massachusetts General Hospital Institute of Health Professionals, Boston, MA; and The University of Texas School of Nursing, Austin, TX. Inquiries should be made to the financial aid officer at one of these schools. The Kemper Foundation is located at Route 22 and Kemper Drive, Long Grove, IL 60049. Telephone (708) 320-2847.

MARINE CORPS SCHOLARSHIP   1, 3, 4
FOUNDATION, INC.

The Foundation, a nonprofit corporation, encourages needy and deserving children of Marines and former Marines to begin or continue their college or vocational/technical education in all fields,

For key to codes showing categories of aid, see page 17.

especially nursing and other health-related fields. Awards range from $500 to $2,500. The applicant must be a senior in high school, a high school graduate, or currently enrolled in a certified college or vocational/technical school. Total family gross income cannot exceed a prescribed limit of $41,000. Applicants must write to the Foundation for application and instructions. Deadline for submission of completed applications is April 1 for the upcoming academic year. For more information, write to: Marine Corps Scholarship Foundation, Inc., P.O. Box 3008, Princeton, NJ 08543-3008. Telephone (609) 921-3534.

MATERNITY CENTER ASSOCIATION FOUNDATION   4, 5

Nurses who have been accepted for study in an ACNM-approved nurse-midwifery program are eligible to apply for a $5,000 grant. Applicants must have received an RN or bachelor's degree in nursing and be pursuing an advanced course in nurse-midwifery. Applications may be submitted, along with a letter of acceptance from the program and a resume, by August 1, 1997. Awards are made once a year. Preference is given to candidates planning to practice in the United States after completing the program. Applications are available from: Maternity Center Association Foundation, 281 Park Ave. South, 5th floor, New York, NY 10010.

NATIONAL ASSOCIATION OF ORTHOPAEDIC NURSES FOUNDATION   3, 4, 5, 6, 7

The National Association of Orthopaedic Nurses Foundation (NAON Foundation) has developed the Awards Program to enhance the education of orthopaedic nurses. Scholarships are available through continuing college education and funding participation in the NAON Annual Congress, as well as other national educational offerings. Funding is also available for research projects and poster presentations specific to orthopaedic nursing. Orthopaedic nurses are encouraged to share their research concepts and clinical practice innovations via abstracts presented at the NAON Annual Congress and to take advantage of these opportunities for funding of their continuing education. Certification scholarships are also available.

The NAON Foundation offers several scholarship awards to qualified students of nursing and professional nurses. These awards are funded either by orthopaedic manufacturers or sister organizations to the NAON Foundation. Awards may be used to assist in acquiring bachelor's or graduate degrees or to advance current knowledge for orthopaedic nurses.

For further information and applications, write to: National Association of Orthopaedic Nurses Foundation, Box 56, Pitman, NJ 08071-0056. Telephone (609) 256-2310.

NATIONAL ASSOCIATION OF PEDIATRIC NURSE ASSOCIATES AND PRACTITIONERS   4, 5

Through the generosity of grants from McNeil Consumer Products Company, NAPNAP will award two annual **NAPNAP/McNeil Scholarships** of $2,000 each to students enrolled in pediatric nurse practitioner programs. Applicants must be RNs with previous work experience in pediatrics; document acceptance at a recognized pediatric nurse practitioner program, either continuing education or master's degree; and demonstrate financial need. Previous formal nurse practitioner education disqualifies the applicant. An applicant's goals and philosophy, expressed in a written statement, must be consistent with those of NAPNAP. Applications are due postmarked by September 30 for spring semester programs and postmarked by May 30 for fall semester programs. Recipients will be notified within eight weeks of the application deadline and recognized at NAPNAP's annual conference. For application forms, write to: National Association of Pediatric Nurse Associates and Practitioners, 1101 Kings Highway North, Suite #206, Cherry Hill, NJ 08034. Telephone (609) 667-1773, fax (609) 667-7187, e-mail 74224.51@compuserve.com, WWW http://www.napnap.org.

NATIONAL CERTIFICATION BOARD: PERIOPERATIVE NURSING, INC. (NCB:PNI) SCHOLARSHIP   3, 5, 7

The NCB:PNI offers scholarships through the Association of Operating Room Nurses (AORN) Foundation to support education, research, scholarships, and fellowships in operating room nursing. The AORN Scholarship Board will be responsible for selecting the yearly NCB:PNI scholarship recipients. For more information on scholarships and other awards available, contact: AORN Scholarships Board, c/o AORN Headquarters, 2170 South Parker Road, Suite 300, Denver, CO 80231.

NATIONAL FOUNDATION FOR INFECTIOUS DISEASES   7

The **National Foundation for Infectious Diseases Young Investigator Matching Grants** award investigators who are beginning their research into infectious diseases and who currently hold full-time junior faculty status at an accredited institution of higher learning. Each award is for $2,000 with $2,000 to be assumed as matching funds from the sponsoring institution. The deadline for application is February 15 for the May 1 award. (Contact the National Foundation for Infectious Diseases in mid-1994 to determine the program's continuance in 1995.)

For more information and application, contact: National Foundation for Infectious Diseases, 4733 Bethesda Avenue, Suite 750, Bethesda, MD 20814. Telephone (301) 656-0003.

NATIONAL INSTITUTE OF NURSING RESEARCH   6, 7
NATIONAL INSTITUTES OF HEALTH
U.S. DEPARTMENT OF HEALTH AND HUMAN SERVICES

The National Institute of Nursing Research (NINR) sponsors the **National Research Service Awards,** which support nurses in predoctoral and postdoctoral research training in specified areas of nursing, biomedical, and behavioral fields. Awards are made to (1) increase the opportunities for qualified nurses to engage in full-time graduate study and research training; (2) prepare professional nurses to conduct independent research, collaborate in interdisciplinary research, and stimulate and guide others in nursing research; (3) promote the availability and utilization of nurses with research training in nursing or the basic and behavioral sciences to function as faculty in schools of nursing; and (4) prepare nurses to conduct scientific inquiry in disciplines that have significance for nursing theory and practice.

For key to codes showing categories of aid, see page 17.

For predoctoral research, applicants must be U.S. citizens or permanent residents, registered nurses with an active license, either a baccalaureate or master's degree in nursing, and be admitted to a doctoral program.

The annual stipend is $10,008. An institutional allowance is also provided to defray tuition and fees, research supplies, equipment, and other related expenses.

For postdoctoral research, applicants must satisfy all requirements previously mentioned, as well as having received a doctorate prior to the beginning date of the proposed fellowship. Applicants must have identified a research project and be accepted by a faculty sponsor who will supervise the training and research.

Postdoctoral stipends are determined by the number of years of relevant experience at the time the award is issued. Relevant experience may include research experience (including industrial), teaching, internship, residency, or full-time studies in a health-related field other than that of the qualifying doctoral degree. Current stipends begin at $19,608 and peak at $32,300. The sponsoring institution may also receive an allowance to defray certain expenses. Fellows are subject to payback obligations. However, this obligation may be met by continuing nursing, biomedical, or behavioral research or teaching after completing the fellowship.

Applications for both pre- and postdoctoral research awards are accepted at any time for inclusion in one of the three annual review cycles beginning April 5, August 5, and December 5.

NINR grants are offered in numerous areas, including, but not limited to: Biobehavioral symptom management, nursing care of persons with HIV, pain assessment and management, issues related to minority populations, prevention and care of low birth weight infants, health behavior in children and adolescents, bioethics and clinical decision making, community based care for chronically ill older persons, and clinical outcomes and nursing practice. Studies which link nursing and the biological sciences are particularly encouraged.

For more information on these and other programs offered by the National Institute of Nursing Research, write: Office of Information and Legislation, National Institute of Nursing Research, National Institutes of Health, Building 31, Room 5B03, Bethesda, MD 20892. Telephone (301) 496-0207. For applications, Extramural Outreach and Information Resources, Office of Extramural

Research, National Institute of Health, 6701 Rockledge Drive, Suite 6095, Bethesda, MD 20892-7910. Telephone (301) 435-0714, fax (301) 480-0525, e-mail asknih@odrockm1.od.nih.gov, WWW http://www.nih.gov.

NATIONAL SOCIETY DAUGHTERS OF THE AMERICAN REVOLUTION   1, 2, 3

The DAR offers a $500 one-time **Caroline E. Holt Nursing Scholarship** award for a student currently enrolled in an accredited undergraduate school of nursing. Criteria include academic excellence, financial need, and commitment to a field of study. Candidates (both male and female) must be sponsored by a local DAR Chapter but do not have to be members of the DAR themselves. For the name and address of the local DAR Chapter, the applicant may contact the Office of the Committees, NSDAR, at the address given below. The award is presented twice a year, with deadlines of February 15 for the April award or August 15 for the October award. For more information and application forms, write to: National Society, Daughters of the American Revolution, Office of the Committees—Scholarships, 1776 D Street, NW, Washington, DC 20006-5392. All written inquiries must be accompanied by a self-addressed, stamped envelope. Telephone (202) 879-3292.

NATIONAL STUDENT NURSES' ASSOCIATION   1, 3

The Foundation of the National Student Nurses' Association will award up to $68,000 in scholarships to undergraduate nursing students in the 1996 Scholarship Program. Scholarships are available to nursing students currently enrolled in nursing or pre-nursing programs in state-approved schools of nursing. Scholarship awards will be based on academic achievement, financial need, and demonstrated commitment to nursing through involvement in student organizations and/or school and community activities related to health care. Applications can be obtained by sending a self-addressed business size envelope with 55 cents postage (2 stamps) to: The Foundation of the National Student Nurses' Association, Inc., 555 West 57th Street, Suite 1327, New York, NY 10019. Applications will be available from September 1997 until January 13, 1998.

For key to codes showing categories of aid, see page 17.

NELLCOR-AMERICAN ASSOCIATION OF 4, 5
CRITICAL-CARE NURSES (AACN) MENTORSHIP GRANT

This award, cosponsored by Nellcor Inc. and AACN, facilitates critical care nursing practice research between a novice and experienced researcher. The novice researcher is a beginning researcher with limited or no research experience in the area of the proposed investigation. The novice researcher is also a registered nurse with current AACN membership. The grant may be used to fund research for an academic degree. The mentor must show strong evidence of research expertise in the proposed area of research to be pursued by the novice investigator. The mentor may not be designated mentor in two consecutive years and may not be conducting research as part of an academic degree. Novice investigator receives up to $10,000. Proposals must be received by February 1.

For further information, please contact: Grants Administrator, American Association of Critical-Care Nurses, 101 Columbia, Aliso Viejo, CA 92656-1491; Application materials and instructions may be requested by calling (800) 899-2226, fax (714) 362-2020.

NIGHTINGALE AWARDS OF PENNSYLVANIA 1, 2

Nightingale Awards of Pennsylvania, a non-profit foundation dedicated to retaining and recruiting nurses in Pennsylvania, invites qualified candidates to apply for scholarships to pursue an education in nursing. Applicants are judged on academic standing, leadership, community service, and commitment to a profession in nursing. Applications must be received by February 1. For further information, contact: Kelly Henning, Hood, Light and Geise, Inc., 509 N. Second Street, Harrisburg, PA 17101. Telephone (717) 234-8091, fax (717) 234-1995.

NURSE ANESTHETIST TRAINEESHIP 5
DIVISION OF NURSING
BUREAU OF HEALTH PROFESSIONS
U.S. DEPARTMENT OF HEALTH AND HUMAN SERVICES

Grants are awarded under this program to accredited public or private nonprofit institutions that provide nurse anesthetist education.

For key to codes showing categories of aid, see page 17.

Trainees must be U.S. citizens or permanent residents; graduates of a state-approved school of nursing and currently licensed as a professional nurse in a U.S. state or territory; and enrolled full-time in a course of study beyond the twelfth month of study in an approved nurse anesthetist program. Applications are made directly to participating institutions that provide nurse anesthesia training, which select trainees and provide financial support. Traineeships provide tuition and fees and stipends of up to $8,800 per year for a maximum of 18 months of study.

For program information, write to: Division of Nursing, Bureau of Health Professions, Health Resources and Services Administration, Room 9-36, Parklawn Building, Nursing Education/Practice Resources Branch, 5600 Fishers Ln., Rockville, MD 20857.

NURSES' EDUCATIONAL FUNDS, INC. 5, 8

Scholarships are available to registered nurses who seek further study in nursing. Men and women qualifying for these awards are expected to study in an NLN-accredited master's program or a nursing or nursing-related doctoral program at a college or university of their choice. The amount and number of awards are determined each year on the basis of availability of funds and qualifications of applicants, ranging from $2,500 to $10,000. Awards are based on academic criteria and potential for leadership in the nursing community. Applicants are required to be citizens of the United States or to have declared official intention of becoming a citizen. In addition, they must be members of a national professional nursing organization. Each scholarship application requires GRE or MAT scores. Deadline for mailing applications is February 1. Application kits are available August 1 and the deadline for completion of all applications is February 1 preceding the academic year for which the awards are made. Scholarship kits are $5 to cover the cost of postage and handling. For more information, write to: Nurses' Educational Funds, Inc., 555 West 57th Street, New York, NY 10019.

ONCOLOGY NURSING FOUNDATION 3, 4, 5, 6, 7

The Oncology Nursing Foundation offers several scholarships to registered nurses with an interest in and commitment to oncology nursing. Forty-One (41) academic scholarships ranging from $2,000 to $3,000 are available. All applicants must have a demonstrated commitment to oncology nursing and applications for each academic year are due by February 1.

The **Roberta Pierce Scofield Undergraduate Scholarship** offers three (3) $2,000 scholarships, the **Immunex Undergraduate Scholarship** offers two (2) $2,000 scholarships, and the **Oncology Nursing Certification Corporation Undergraduate Scholarship** offers ten (10) $2,000 scholarships to RNs who have demonstrated a commitment to cancer nursing and are currently enrolled as either full-time or part-time students in an undergraduate nursing degree program in an NLN-accredited school of nursing.

The **Pharmacia & UpJohn, Inc. Graduate Scholarship** offers one (1) $3,000 scholarship, the **Glaxo Wellcome Oncology Graduate Scholarship** offers two (2) $3,000 scholarships, the **Oncology Nursing Certification Corporation** offers two (2) $3,000 graduate scholarships, and the **Oncology Nursing Foundation Graduate Scholarship** offers nine (9) $3,000 scholarships to RNs who have demonstrated a commitment to cancer nursing and are currently enrolled as either full-time or part-time students in a graduate nursing degree program in an NLN-accredited school of nursing. The program must have application to oncology nursing.

The **Ann Olson Doctoral Scholarship** offers one (1) $3,000 scholarship, the **Thomas Jordan Doctoral Scholarship** offers one (1) $3,000 scholarship, and the **Oncology Nursing Foundation Doctoral Scholarship** offers three (3) $3,000 scholarships to RNs who have demonstrated a commitment to cancer nursing and are currently enrolled in or applying as either full-time or part-time students to a doctoral nursing degree or related program for study of nursing applicable to oncology nursing.

For more information on these and other scholarship programs, write to: Oncology Nursing Foundation, 501 Holiday Drive, Pittsburgh, PA 15220-2749.

PARTNERSHIPS FOR TRAINING   1, 7

This program has been established to address shortages of primary care practitioners in medically-underserved areas. The program will support the development of innovative regional educational models for nurse practioners (NPs), certified nurse-midwives (CNMs), and physician assistants (PAs) that emphasize training these new professionals within their own communities. The program is intended to spark partnerships among schools, employers of health professionals, and public and private funders to facilitate the program development and policy changes needed to foster more supportive practice environments for these clinicians.

To receive a brochure describing application guidelines, write: Communications Department, The Robert Wood Johnson Foundation, College Road, P.O. Box 2316, Princeton, NJ 08543-2316.

PROFESSIONAL NURSE TRAINEESHIPS   5
DIVISION OF NURSING
BUREAU OF HEALTH PROFESSIONS
U.S. DEPARTMENT OF HEALTH AND HUMAN SERVICES

Traineeships are awarded to currently licensed professional nurses through grants to (1) public or private nonprofit institutions providing master's and doctoral degree programs to educate nurses to serve as nurse practitioners, nurse educators, or other nursing specialists in medically underserved communities especially; and (2) public or private nonprofit schools of nursing and other entities to educate nurses as nurse-midwives. Trainees are selected by participating training institutions in accordance with the institution's admission policies and the purpose of the traineeship program. Traineeships provide for tuition and fees as established by the training institution and stipends up to $8,800 per year for a maximum of 36 months of study. Candidates must be U.S. citizens, or lawfully admitted to the United States for permanent residence; graduates of a state-approved school of nursing; currently licensed as RNs; and able to enroll for full-time study. Awards are made by participating schools, which includes most graduate nursing programs. Traineeship applications must be made directly to the school, not to the Division of Nursing. For program information, write to: Division of Nursing, Bureau of Health Professions, Health Resources and Services Administration, Room 9-36, Parklawn Bldg., Rockville, MD 20857, Attention: Nursing Practice Resources Section. Telephone (301) 443-5763.

For key to codes showing categories of aid, see page 17.

REHABILITATION NURSING CERTIFICATION   3
BOARD'S BSN SCHOLARSHIP

The Rehabilitation Nursing Certification Board (RNCB) of the Association of Rehabilitation Nurses (ARN) is offering a $1,000 scholarships to ARN members who are pursuing a bachelor of science in nursing degree (BSN); the deadline for applying is June 1. Eligibility requirements include current ARN membership status, current enrollment in good standing in a baccalaureate program, a minimum of 2 years rehabilitation nursing experience, and current practice in rehabilitation nursing. For application materials, please contact the RNCB office at 4700 W. Lake Avenue, Glenview, IL 60025. Telephone (800) 229-7530 or (847) 1375-4710.

THE ROBERT WOOD JOHNSON FOUNDATION   7

The Robert Wood Johnson Foundation offers several distinct grant programs for research, traineeships, and postdoctoral work.

Colleagues in Caring: Regional Collaboratives for Nursing Work Force Development is a nationally competitive grants program. It is to help nursing schools, hospitals, and other nursing service institutions initiate concerted work force development systems within their regions. The systems would feature formal consortia among regional nursing schools designed to: (1) enable individual nurses to pursue a continuum of education throughout their professional careers, from the LPN to the doctorate; (2) prepare RNs to meet all of the regional nursing care needs (acute, long-term, chronic, primary care, and public health); and (3) develop a regional cadre of RNs for leadership roles as clinicians, educators, and service managers. For further information, please contact: Mary F. Rapson, PhD, RN, Colleagues in Caring: Regional Collaboratives for Nursing Work Force Development, American Association of Colleges of Nursing, One Dupont Circle, NW, Suite 530, Washington, DC 20036. Telephone (202) 496-1095, fax (202) 496-1093.

Partnerships for Training: Regional Education Systems for Nurse Practitioners, Certified Nurse-Midwives, and Physician Assistants is designed to address shortages of primary care practitioners in medically-underserved areas. Partnerships for Training will support the development of innovative regional education

For key to codes showing categories of aid, see page 17.

models for nurse practitioners (NP), certified nurse-midwives (CNMs), and physician assistants (PAs) that emphasize training these new professionals, and public and private funders to facilitate the program development and policy changes needed to foster more supportive practice environments for these clinicians. For further information, please contact: Jean Johnson-Pawlson, Partnerships for Training, Association for Academic Health Centers, 1616 "P" Street, NW, Suite 400, Washington, DC 20036. Telephone (202) 797-6544, fax (202) 797-6546.

Tobacco Policy Research and Evaluation Program has been established to provide useful information for policymakers concerned about reducing tobacco use in the United States. Researchers from policy sciences will be expected to assess and evaluate the best strategies for reducing the onset of tobacco use, and to provide a full understanding of the advantages, disadvantages, and impact of public and private policy alternatives. To receive a brochure describing application guidelines, write: Communications Department, The Robert Wood Johnson Foundation, College Road, P.O. Box 2316, Princeton, NJ 08543-2316.

ROBERT W. WOODRUFF FELLOWSHIPS IN NURSING

1, 3, 4, 5

The Nell Hodgson Woodruff School of Nursing of Emory University offers several graduate fellowships to exemplary individuals dedicated to the field of nursing. Fellowships cover full tuition toward master's degrees in any one of 12 areas of nursing specialization. Applicant criteria include outstanding academic achievement, superior leadership, creativity in school and community, and significant vision for and commitment to the profession. Applicants must be nominated by either the dean of their school of nursing or the director of nursing of their current employer. Nominations are due not later than December 15, and completed applications must be received no later than February 1. Merit Scholarships based on academic achievement are also available. For more information on available scholarships, write to: Office of Student Affairs, Nell Hodgson Woodruff School of Nursing, Emory University, Atlanta, GA 30322. Telephone (404) 727-7980 or (800) 222-3879, WWW http://www .emory.edu/WHSC/NURSING.

For key to codes showing categories of aid, see page 17.

SIGMA THETA TAU INTERNATIONAL   3, 4, 5, 7
HONOR SOCIETY OF NURSING

Sigma Theta Tau International offers grant programs for qualified nurse applicants who have received formal preparation for research at the graduate level. Candidates for awards are required to be registered nurses, to have received a master's degree, have a well-defined research project pertinent to nursing, and be ready to start or already be in the process of the research. Preference will be given to Sigma Theta Tau members, other attributes being equal. Allocation of funds is based on the quality of the proposed research, past performance and future promise of the applicant, and the research budget. The **Sigma Theta Tau Small Grant** encourages pilot, multidisciplinary, and international research. Ten to fifteen grants are offered with a maximum amount of $3,000 awarded to an applicant. Applicants are required to be received by March 1. The **American Nurses' Foundation Grant** encourages research on a clinical topic of reference. One grant for $6,000 is offered. Applications are required to be received by May 1. The **Mead Johnson Nutritionals Perinatal Grant** encourages research on perinatal issues spanning the prenatal period through the first year of life. Research topics may include, but are not limited to, low- and high-risk maternal and neonatal care practices and innovative patient care delivery systems. One grant for the sum of $10,000 is the maximum amount to be awarded to an applicant. Application is required to be received by June 1. The **Sigma Theta Tau/American Association of Critical Care Nurses Critical-Care Grant (AACN)** encourages research on critical care nursing practice. One grant for $10,000 is the maximum amount awarded. Applications are required by October 1. The **Sigma Theta Tau/Oncology Nursing Society Grant (ONS)** encourages research on an oncology clinically oriented topic. One grant for $10,000 is the maximum amount to be awarded. Applications are required by December 1. **Sigma Theta Tau International/Glaxo Wellcome Prescriptive Practice Grant** encourages research on prescribing practices of advanced practice nurses. Although funds are provided by Glaxo Wellcome Inc., preference will be given to Sigma Theta Tau members. **Sigma Theta Tau International/Glaxo Wellcome New Investigator Grants** encourage research focusing on nursing issues related to medication and medication administration. The Sigma Theta Tau International/Glaxo New Investigator Research Grant will award $3,000 to a nurse practicing full-time in an adult clinical setting. Applications are required by October 1. For further information on these grant programs, contact: Program Department, Sigma Theta Tau, 550 West North Street, Indianapolis, IN 46202. Telephone (317) 634-8171.

The **Sigma Theta Tau International/ENA Foundation Grant** provides funds for two recipients in the amount of $3,000 each for research to advance the specialized practice of emergency nursing. Priority will be given to studies which relate to ENA Research Initiatives. These include: mechanisms to assure effective, efficient, and quality emergency nursing care delivery systems; factors effecting emergency nursing practice; factors effecting health care cost; productivity, and market forces to emergency services; ways to enhance health promotion and injury prevention; and mechanisms to assure quality and cost effective educational programs for emergency nursing. Applications are required by March 1. For further information, write: ENA Foundation, 216 Higgins Road, Park Ridge, Il 60068-5735. Telephone (847) 698-9400, ext. 3350 or fax (847) 698-9407 or on the WWW http://www.ena.org.

STUDENT LOAN PROGRAM (NURSING) 1, 2, 3
U.S. DEPARTMENT OF HEALTH AND HUMAN SERVICES

This program is intended to assist students achieve careers in nursing by providing long-term, low-interest-rate loans to help meet costs of education. Students may borrow $2,500 for an academic year, $4,000 for each of the final two years, or the amount of financial need, whichever is the lesser. The total amount of a student's loan for all years may not exceed $13,000. For more information on the Student Loan Program (Nursing), contact the Director of Student Financial Aid at the school where you intend to apply for admission or where you are enrolled.

SUBSTANCE ABUSE AND MENTAL HEALTH   5, 6, 7
SERVICES ADMINISTRATION FACULTY
DEVELOPMENT GRANTS FOR PREVENTING
ALCOHOL, TOBACCO, AND OTHER DRUG USE

These grants are offered to nursing/health science institutions to support training in substance abuse prevention for health care professionals in academic posts. Only accredited schools of nursing/health science need apply. The grant application is due May 24.

For more information contact: Dr. Lucille Perez, Medical Nursing Grants, Office of the Director, Substance Abuse and Mental Health Services Administration, 5600 Fishers Ln., Rockwall II Bldg., Rockville, MD 20857. Telephone (301) 443-5276; or Mary Lou Dent, Acting Grants Management Officer, Center for Substance Abuse Prevention, Public Health Service (301) 443-3958.

U.S. PUBLIC HEALTH SERVICE   3, 7
DIVISION OF SCHOLARSHIPS AND
LOAN REPAYMENTS

For fiscal year 1997, Nursing Education Loan Repayment Program (NELRP) Funds are available for qualified applicants. The funds will repay amounts borrowed for tuition, fees, educational expenses, and reasonable living expenses. Registered nurses employed in health care facilities in geographic areas with a critical shortage of nurses are given preference. Eligible health care facilities include Indian Health Service health centers, Native Hawaiian health centers, public hospitals, migrant health centers, community health centers, and public or nonprofit health facilities. Funds received will depend on availability and the amount of time individual nurses agree to work in an eligible health care facility: for two years of work under the NELRP, 60 percent of the verifiable loan balance is repaid; for three years of work, 85 percent of the verifiable loan balance is repaid. To apply, write to: Bureau of Primary Health Care, Division of Scholarships and Loan Repayments, Attention: NELRP, 4350 East West Highway, 10th Floor, Bethesda, MD 20814. Telephone (301) 594-4400.

For key to codes showing categories of aid, see page 17.

UNIVERSITY OF PENNSYLVANIA SCHOOL 1, 3, 5, 6, 7
OF NURSING

The Alex Hillman Family Foundation Scholarship Program offers support to undergraduate and graduate students attending the University of Pennsylvania School of Nursing.

Undergraduate students receive partial tuition support over four years in exchange for a two year work commitment in any New York City hospital after graduation. Graduate students receive partial tuition support for one year in exchange for a one year work commitment in a New York City hospital, home or health care agency.

For more information on the program write to: University of Pennsylvania School of Nursing, ATTN: Gina Marziani, 420 Guardian Drive, Nursing Education Building, Philadelphia, PA 19104-6096. Telephone (215) 898-8285.

WESTERN REGIONAL GRADUATE PROGRAM 5

The Western Regional Graduate Program has more than 100 master's and doctoral programs in 35 institutions in which residents of 14 states (Alaska, Arizona, Colorado, Hawaii, Idaho, Montana, Nevada, New Mexico, North Dakota, Oregon, South Dakota, Utah, Washington, and Wyoming) may enroll at resident tuition. For graduate study in nursing, nine programs are currently available: Nursing (PhD), University of Arizona, Tucson, AZ; Nursing (PhD), University of Colorado Health Sciences Center, Denver, CO; Rural Nursing (MSN), Montana State University, Billings, MT; Nursing Science (PhD), Oregon Health Sciences University, Portland, OR; Nursing and Latin American Studies (MS, Nursing, MA, Latin American Studies) University of New Mexico, Albuquerque, NM; Nursing (PhD), Clinical Nursing Informatics (MS), and Oncology Clinical Nurse Specialist (MS), University of Utah, Salt Lake City, UT; and Rural Health Nursing (MS), University of Wyoming, Laramie, WY. Students may apply directly to the program of interest and must identify themselves as "WICHE WRGP" applicants. For more information and/or brochure, write: Western Regional Graduate Program, WICHE, P.O. Box 9752, Boulder, CO 80301-9752. Telephone (303) 541-0210.

For key to codes showing categories of aid, see page 17.

WOUND, OSTOMY, AND CONTINENCE   4, 5
NURSES SOCIETY (WOCN)

Scholarships are offered by the WOCN four times a year to nurses who wish to pursue a career in providing care to persons with abdominal stomas, fecal and urinary diversions, draining wounds, pressure ulcers, or incontinence. Applicants must hold a current RN license, possess a baccalaureate degree with a major in nursing, and have a minimum of two years clinical nursing experience. Awards are based upon personal merit and financial need to assist individuals in studying at any of the schools accredited for enterostomal therapy, wound, ostomy and continence care nursing education in the United States. Applicants must be accepted into an educational program before applying for scholarship funding.

Scholarships are also available to enterostomal therapy nurses who are working toward an advanced degree in nursing. Applicants must be currently seeking a baccalaureate, master's, or doctoral degree in nursing in an NLN-accredited program; a graduate of an accredited WOCN enterostomal therapy nursing education program; board certified in enterostomal therapy nursing; a current and active member of the WOCN; and have at least two years of ET nursing experience within the past five years. A 3.0 grade point average is required. All applicants are selected by blind review based upon merit, financial need, and compliance with the basic eligibility criteria.

For additional information, write to: Wound, Ostomy, and Continence Nurses Society (WOCN), 1550 S. Coast Highway, Suite 201, Laguna Beach, CA 92651. Telephone (888) 224-WOCN, fax (714) 376-3456, WWW http://www.wocn.org.

For key to codes showing categories of aid, see page 17.

Aid for Minority Students

This chapter focuses on scholarships that are awarded specifically to minority students who wish to pursue a career in nursing and, in some cases, health-care-related fields. (Some of the scholarships listed in this section are open to applications from non-minority students as well; but in reality, because funds for aid are always limited, the number of awards granted to such non-minority applicants is very small.) Minority students are encouraged to read about all the scholarships and loans described in this book as well as the ones listed in this chapter.

Of course, there are also many sources of aid for minority students that are not specifically related to nursing. Several of the publications listed in the Resources section have special sections on aid for minority students. Two books—*Directory of Special Programs for Minority Group Members* and *Financial Aid for Minorities in Health Fields*—list both general and specialty programs that are targeted at members of minority groups, as well as highlight general programs that are open to all but may have special provisions or emphases for minority students. In addition to the aid mentioned here for American Indian students, many states and tribes have special programs. Listings are available from the Indian Fellowship Program, U.S. Department of Education, Office of Elementary and Secondary Education, Washington, DC 20202.

AMERICAN INDIAN GRADUATE CENTER   4, 5, 7, 8

The American Indian Graduate Center announces the availability of graduate (master's and doctoral) fellowships in nursing and other health-related fields for American Indian and Alaskan Native students from federally recognized tribes. Fellowship eligibility also requires that the applicant be in need of financial aid *after* exhausting available aid at the institution which he or she attends. Fellowships are based on each applicant's unmet financial need. Application deadline is June 2, 1997 for the 1997–1998 academic year. Application packets are available from: American Indian Graduate Center, 4520 Montgomery Boulevard, NE, Suite 1-B, Albuquerque, NM 87109. Telephone (505) 881-4584.

AMERICAN NURSES' ASSOCIATION CLINICAL   6, 8
TRAINING PROGRAM FELLOWSHIPS

Funded by the National Institutes of Health and by the Center for Mental Health Services, these programs aim to increase and improve mental health treatment and research on issues of importance to ethnic and racial minority populations. Fellowships are awarded to nurses for the pursuit of doctoral degrees in psychiatric and mental health nursing or behavioral science that will help them prepare for careers in the delivery of nursing to ethnic and racial minority groups. The Clinical fellowship is awarded for one year but can be renewed for up to three years. The Research fellowship is also awarded annually but can be renewed for up to five years. The application deadline is January 15, and the maximum fellowship award is $10,008. For more information, write: American Nurses' Association, Ethnic/Racial Minority Fellowship Programs, 600 Maryland Ave., SW, Suite 100W, Washington, DC 20024. Telephone (202) 651-7244.

AMERICAN NURSES' ASSOCIATION   4, 6, 8
ETHNIC/RACIAL MINORITY FELLOWSHIP PROGRAMS

Designed for, but not limited to, ethnic minority registered nurses, the **Registered Nurse Research Fellowship Program** provides support for psychiatric nurses to pursue doctoral study in the behavioral sciences, and the **Clinical Fellowship Program** provides support in clinical psychiatric nursing. The programs are intended to increase the number of minority nurses in psychiatric nursing with

For key to codes showing categories of aid, see page 17.

doctoral degrees in mental health research and in clinical psychiatric and mental health nursing. The deadline for applications is January 15 of each year for funding to begin in September of the same year. Each fellow may receive up to $10,950 a year, which includes an allowance for tuition and stipend. Awards are paid directly to each fellow, and are renewable annually (up to three years), contingent upon satisfactory academic performance and renewed grant funding. The programs are funded by the Minority Research Resources Branch, National Institute of Mental Health. In exchange for monies received, clinical fellows must agree to provide or engage in payback services which meet guidelines set by the Alcohol, Drug Abuse, and Mental Health Administration for a period of time equal to the period of support. For information, write to: American Nurses Association, Ethnic/Racial Minority Fellowship Programs, 600 Maryland Ave., SW, Suite 100W, Washington, DC 20024-2571. Telephone (202) 651-7244, ext. 122, fax (202) 651-7007.

ASSOCIATION ON AMERICAN INDIAN AFFAIRS, INC. SCHOLARSHIP PROGRAM

1, 3, 4, 8

Since 1923, the Association on American Indian Affairs has been helping Native American people and their communities in meeting educational challenges. They offer several scholarships for the Native American Indian.

A new scholarship program, **Displaced Homemaker Scholarships,** has been established for mid-life homemakers, both men and women, who are unable to fulfill their educational goals. The scholarship program will identify eligible women and men who would not otherwise be able to finish their education and support them for up to three years with funds for their special needs as heads of household, as single parents, or as displaced homemakers. The **Displaced Homemaker Program** will augment the usual and expected financial sources of educational money to assist those students to gain degrees, child care, transportation, and some basic living expenses.

The **Adolph Van Pelt Scholarships** for undergraduate and gr~ uate students are in amounts ranging from $500 to $800. Th~ gram is based on financial need and merit. Grants, awarded in August, are paid directly to accredited educational insti~ monies can be used for tuition, books, and other aca

For key to codes showing categories of aid

expenses. The grant is renewable for up to four years of support toward any one degree. Each year the grant is renewed with $100 added to the scholarship. Applications are due June 1st of each year; recipients are notified by June 30th.

The **Emergency Aid and Health Professions Scholarships** for American Indian and Alaskan Native students offer amounts ranging from $50 to $300 during the academic school year. The program is for full-time **undergraduate students only,** based on financial need, and is limited by the availability of scholarship funds. Students may only receive one scholarship per academic year. Scholarships are available from September 1st through June 1st of the academic year.

From July 1st through September 13th of each academic year applications will be accepted for the **Sequoyah Graduate Fellowship** for American Indian and Alaskan Native graduate students. The Fellowship provides a one-year, $1,500 unrestricted stipend. There is no subject matter requirement; fellowships are awarded to American Indians and Alaskan Natives who are pursuing graduate degrees in many diverse fields. For more information, contact: Association on American Indian Affairs, Inc., 245 Fifth Avenue, Suite 1801, New York, NY 10016-8728. Telephone (212) 689-3720.

FOUNDATION OF THE NATIONAL STUDENT NURSES' ASSOCIATION

(1, 3, 8)

Breakthrough to Nursing Scholarships are offered annually to ethnic/minority students of color for basic nursing education. In making awards, extra credit goes to members of the National Student Nurses' Association, but all students are eligible for these awards. Applications are available until January 15. Deadline for applications is February 1. For information and applications, send a self-addressed business-size envelope with 55¢ postage to: Foundation of the National Student Nurses' Association, 555 West 57th Street, Suite 1327, New York, NY 10019. Telephone (212) 581-2211.

HEADLANDS INDIAN HEALTH CAREER GRANTS 1, 2, 8

This grant was established to increase the science and math background d communication skills of Native American students interested in a career in the health professions. Applicants must be (1) in the senior year of high school with a minimum grade point average of 2.5, or in the first year of college, and (2) credited with at least 2 years of algebra and 2 science courses. Each awardee is provided free room and board, tuition, a $500 stipend, and air transportation to an eight-week enhancement program held during the summer of each year. For more information and application, contact: Headlands Indian Health Career BSEB-200, P.O. Box 26901, Oklahoma City, OK 75190. Telephone (405) 271-2250. Application deadline: March 1.

HEALTH RESOURCES AND SERVICES ADMINISTRATION NURSING EDUCATION OPPORTUNITIES FOR THE DISADVANTAGED PROJECT GRANTS

7

This program is intended to provide financial assistance to eligible schools of nursing and other applicants to meet the costs of special projects to increase nursing education opportunities for individuals from disadvantaged backgrounds. Funds may be used for salaries of personnel specifically employed for the project; consultant fees; supplies and equipment necessary to conduct the project; essential travel expenses; and other expenses related to the project. Indirect costs are allowed for administrative costs, limited to 8 percent of direct costs. Grants may be made for up to three-year project periods and may be renewed competitively for an additional two years. Public and non-profit private schools of nursing and other public or nonprofit private entities are eligible. For further information, contact: Dr. Helen Lotsikas, Division of Nursing, John Westcott, Grants Management Officer, Health Resources and Services Administration, 5600 Fishers Ln., Parklawn Bldg., Rockville, MD 20857. Telephone (301) 443-6193 or (301) 443-6880.

HIGHER EDUCATION GRANT   1, 2, 3, 5, 8
PROGRAM FOR INDIANS

This program provides financial aid to eligible Indian students, based on demonstrated financial need, to attend nationally accredited institutions of higher education. Grants cover tuition, required fees, books, and other expenses directly related to college attendance, and are supplemental to campus-based aid. To be eligible for this program, an individual must be "a member of a federally recognized tribe."

For more information, an eligible applicant should first contact his or her tribe or agency/area education office. If the applicant does not have this information, he or she may contact the Branch of Post-Secondary Education, Office of Indian Education Programs, 1849 C Street, NW - MS-3512-MIB, Washington, DC 20240. Telephone (202) 219-1127.

INDEPENDENCE FOUNDATION GRANTS PROGRAM   7

The foundation currently has two major areas of interest: independent schools of nursing and health care facilities. The primary goal is to address the nursing and health care needs of those living in poverty and the nursing education of minorities and women in the Delaware Valley region and rural Pennsylvania. A brief letter outlining a proposed project is a prerequisite to a formal application. Applications are due September 30th. For further information, contact: Theodore Warner Jr., President, Independence Foundation, 1345 Chestnut St., 2500 Philadelphia National Bank Bldg., Philadelphia, PA 19107-3493. Telephone (215) 563-8105, fax (215) 563-6483.

INDIAN EDUCATION FELLOWSHIP PROGRAM   5, 8
U.S. DEPARTMENT OF EDUCATION

This program provides fellowships to enable American Indians, Eskimos, Aleuts, or other Alaskan Natives to pursue, among other courses of study, a postbaccalaureate degree in nursing. Individual applicants must be accepted or currently enrolled at an institution of higher learning and demonstrate financial need.

For key to codes showing categories of aid, see page 17.

The priorities allocated to the various fields supported by this program and the amount of funds allocated to each vary from year to year. In the 1993–1994 academic year, fellowships from $600 to $24,000 were awarded. Fellowships may be awarded up to the amount of the student's need, taking into account resources, including other sources of financial aid. Funds may be provided for tuition and required fees, stipend, dependency allowance, books, and, if necessary, research and travel expenses. Financial need and the applicant's resources are taken into account in determining the amount of the award.

Fellowships are allocated for a period not to exceed two years and on the basis of (1) academic record and leadership potential, (2) commitment to the field, and (3) financial need.

For more information and application, contact: Dr. John Derby, Chief, Indian Fellowship Program, Office of Indian Education, U.S. Department of Education, Room 2177, FOB 6, 400 Maryland Avenue, SW, Washington, DC 20202-6335. Telephone (202) 401-1902.

INDIAN HEALTH SERVICE SCHOLARSHIP PROGRAM
1, 2, 3, 4, 5, 8
DHHS, PHS, INDIAN HEALTH SERVICE
U.S. DEPARTMENT OF HEALTH AND HUMAN SERVICES

American Indian and Alaska Native nursing students are eligible to apply for two scholarship programs conducted by the Indian Health Service: The Health Professions Preparatory Scholarship Program and the Health Professions Scholarship Program.

The **Health Professions Preparatory Scholarship Program** provides financial assistance for American Indian and Alaska Native students to enroll in compensatory courses (required to improve science, mathematics, or other basic skills) or preprofessional courses, such as a prenursing course, that will qualify them for admission to a health professions program. Applicants must intend to serve the Indian people in their health profession upon completing their professional education. Funding is up to two years.

The **Health Professions Scholarship Program** provides assistance to enrolled members of Federally Recognized Tribes who are enrolled in an NLN-accredited associate, baccalaureate, or master's degree nursing program. Funding is available for up to four years.

For key to codes showing categories of aid, see page 17.

Applicants must sign a contract entering into a service obligation to provide health services in full-time clinical practice with (1) the Indian Health Service; (2) A program conducted under a contract entered into under the Indian Self-Determination Act (P.L. 93-638); (3) A program assisted under Title V of the Indian Health Care Improvement Act (P.L. 94-437); or, (4) The private practice of the nursing profession if such practice is situated in a health professional shortage area and addresses the health care needs of a substantial number of Indians.

Applicants for scholarships can be either full-time or part-time study. Criteria include academic performance, faculty-employer evaluations (recommendations), and student narrative indicating reason for requesting the scholarship. Benefits include full payment of tuition and mandatory fees and a monthly stipend for living expenses ($828 for school year 1996–1997). A lump sum is given for other expenses such as books and travel, but not daily commuting.

The deadline for applications is April 1 of every year. Recipients of scholarships are notified by July 1 of each year. Number of awards are based on the funding available for that year.

For further information contact: The IHS Scholarship Program, Twinbrook Metro Plaza Building, Suite 100A, 12300 Twinbrook Parkway, Rockville, MD 20852.

Indian Health Service Loan Repayment Awards are currently offered to ensure an adequate supply of trained health professionals for Indian Health Service (IHS) facilities. Applicants sign contractual agreements with the Secretary for two years and fulfill their agreements through full-time clinical practice at an IHS facility or approved Indian health program. In return, the LRP will repay up to $30,000 a year for two years of the applicant's eligible health professionals educational loans (undergraduate and graduate) for tuition expenses. Applicants must have a degree in a health profession, and be eligible for, or hold, an appointment as a commissioned officer in the Regular or Reserve Corps of the Public Health Service (PHS); be eligible for selection for civilian service in the Regular or Reserve Corps of the PHS; meet the professional standards for civil service employment in the IHS; or be employed in an Indian health program without service obligation.

Eligible applicants also include health professionals in postgraduate training, or in their final year of health professions school.

For key to codes showing categories of aid, see page 17.

Qualified government and commercial educational loans are those obtained for pursuit of health professions education.

Priority for selection will be given to: Osteopathic physicians certified in or eligible in any specialty provided that the IHS has a need for that specialty; and allopathic physicians may be funded only if they are board certified, eligible in family medicine, internal medicine, pediatrics, geriatric medicine, obstetrics and gynecology, and psychiatry; nurse practitioners, public health nurses, registered nurses, nurse anesthetists, and certified nurse midwives.

Monthly application deadlines are scheduled for the Friday of the second full week of each month. Applicants selected for participation in the fiscal year (FY) 1997 program cycle must begin their service period no later than September 30, 1997.

For further information, write or call the LRP at: Indian Health Service, Loan Repayment Program, Twinbrook Metro Plaza—Suite 100, 12300 Twinbrook Parkway, Rockville, MD 20852. Telephone (301) 443-3396.

The **Nurse Education Program** has been established to recruit and fund qualified nursing students at six schools of nursing that offer associate, baccalaureate and master's programs: Salish Kootenai Community College, School of Nursing, St. Ignatius, MT; University of North Dakota, School of Nursing, Grand Forks, ND; Arizona State University, School of Nursing, Tempe, AZ; State University of New York, School of Nursing, Buffalo, NY; Oglala Lakota Community College, School of Nursing, Pine Ridge, SD; and University of Wisconsin, School of Nursing, Eau Claire, WI. The cap amount for this award is $15,500 per student. All applications must be made through the schools listed above.

For more information on the program briefly discussed here, contact the school in which you are interested.

NATIONAL ASSOCIATION OF HISPANIC NURSES
1, 2, 3, 4, 5, 6, 8

The National Association of Hispanic Nurses promotes leadership and educational advancement for Hispanic/Latina(o) nurses to meet the health care needs of the Hispanic/Latino community. For more information on scholarships and awards, write to: President,

National Association of Hispanic Nurses, 1501 16th St., NW, Washington, DC 20036.

The Ildaura Murillo-Rohde Scholarships was established to offset tuition costs for outstanding Hispanic associate, diploma, baccalaureate, or graduate students. Recipients will be selected on the basis of potential to graduate, current academic standing in an accredited school of nursing (minimum 2.5 GPA), potential for contribution to the profession, and financial need. The amount awarded each year depends on the availability of funds. An applicant must be currently enrolled in an accredited school of nursing and be a US citizen or legal resident of the United States, Puerto Rico, or the US territories. Applications are due by June 1. For further information, please contact: Vice President, National Association of Hispanic Nurses, 9615 Coolbrook, San Antonio, TX 78250.

NATIONAL BLACK NURSES ASSOCIATION 1, 2, 3, 7, 8

The National Black Nurses Association offers several scholarships. The **Lauranne Sams Scholarship Award** is for nursing students enrolled in current programs who meet the following criteria: academic excellence, professional commitment, personal integrity, active involvement in the African-American community, and demonstration of need. Other scholarships are dedicated to generic nursing students and RNs/LVNs completing their baccalaureate degrees. Candidates must be members of NBNA and active members of a local chapter (if one exists in the area). The deadline for submissions is April 15.

The **Mayo Foundation Scholarships** is for undergraduate and graduate nurses enrolled at any level in a nursing program. Awards range from $500 to $2,000. Each application must be approved by the applicant's local NBNA chapter. Candidates may submit applications directly to the NBNA if no local chapter exists in the area. Scholarship winners will be notified by July 1, and the awards are presented at the association's annual conference in August. Applications and information may be obtained by writing to the office. Applications are due April 15. For the **Oates Memorial Scholarship**, please follow the same directions as for the Mayo Foundation Scholarships described above.

For key to codes showing categories of aid, see page 17.

For more information and application forms, write: National Black Nurses' Association, P.O. Box 1823, Washington, DC 20003-1823. Telephone (202) 393-6870. Applicant must send a self-addressed, business-sized, stamped (78 cents) envelop for application processing.

NATIONAL CAUCUS AND CENTER ON BLACK   8
AGED LONG-TERM CARE MINORITY TRAINING
AND DEVELOPMENT PROGRAM

The program provides on-the-job training, licensing preparation, and appropriate in-service training for minorities interested in administrative positions in nursing home, congregate housing, and life care facilities. Approximately seven people are supported at any one time. The internships are awarded for a 12-month period throughout the United States. Applicants must be ethnic minorities with a bachelor's or master's degree in gerontology, social work, health care, or business or public administration with a minimum of two years of full-time work experience in a nursing home or life care facility. Applicants are given a $1,200 monthly stipend plus benefits for up to one year. Proposals are due September 1. For further information, contact: Minority Training and Development Program, National Caucus and Center on Black Aged, 1424 K Street, NW, Ste 500, Washington, DC 20005. Telephone (202) 637-8400.

NATIONAL INSTITUTE OF MENTAL HEALTH   8

The NIMH offers several fellowships and grants in support of minority nurse research. **The Minority Research Fellowships in Psychology and in Mental Health Nursing** encourage applications to support the development and training of individuals in doctoral programs in psychology and mental health nursing to enable them to undertake productive careers in scientific investigations related to mental health and mental illness. A minority research fellowship grant may be made for a period of up to five years.

The Institutional Clinical Training Grants for Racial/Ethnic Minority and Disadvantaged Students are designed to support recruitment and education of racial/ethnic minority and disadvantaged students to become professionals in the core mental health disciplines of social work, psychiatric nursing, psychology, psychiatry, and marriage and family therapy. Any trainee who receives a clinical traineeship in one of the core disciplines, in an established training program for a period of 180 days or more, must pay back a period of obligated service equal to the length of the traineeship. Accredited and/or approved departments/divisions in the mental health core disciplines of psychiatric nursing, psychiatry, psychology, social work, and marriage and family therapy in US colleges or universities, including territories and possessions, are eligible. Applications may be for predoctoral and/or postdoctoral training in any of these fields. For further information contact: Dr. Stephen Koslow, Director, Division of Neuroscience and Behavioral Science, National Institute of Mental Health, 5600 Fishers Ln., Parklawn Bldg., Rockville, MD 20857. Telephone (301) 443-3563.

The Underrepresented Minority Nurses Research Fellowships are designed to support the development and training of underrepresented minority individuals in doctoral programs in mental health nursing to enable them to undertake productive careers in scientific investigations related to mental health and mental disorders. A letter of intent is due by August 1, and the application is due by September 17. For more information, contact: Dr. George Niederehe, Division of Clinical and Treatment Research, National Institute of Mental Health, 5600 Fishers Ln., Parklawn Bldg., Rockville, MD 20857. Telephone (301) 443-3264, fax (301) 594-6783, e-mail gniedere@nih.gov or NIH grant line: (301) 402-2221, the NIH gopher(gopher.nih.gov), and the NIH website (http://www.nih.gov).

NATIONAL SOCIETY OF THE   1, 2, 3, 4, 5, 8
COLONIAL DAMES OF AMERICA

The National Society of the Colonial Dames of America provides a small number of scholarship grants to assist students of American Indian heritage who are studying nursing. These grants are for $500–$1,000 per year, and are to be used for tuition or for expenses applicable to the student's approved program.

The candidates must be: (1) an American Indian (who is *not* a recipient of an Indian Health Services Scholarship); (2) a nursing student already enrolled in a nursing program; (3) in need of financial assistance; and (4) working toward a career goal directly related to the needs of the Indian people.

The student must maintain a satisfactory academic record and be recommended by his or her counselor or other school official. Awards can be given for consecutive years to an individual recipient. For further information and an application, contact: The National Society of The Colonial Dames of America, Indian Nurse Scholarship Awards, Mrs. Henry Eugene Trotter, Consultant, 3064 Luvan Blvd., deBordieu, Georgetown, SC 29440.

NEW YORK LIFE FOUNDATION SCHOLARSHIP PROGRAM FOR WOMEN IN THE HEALTH PROFESSIONS

1, 2, 3, 4, 5, 8

These scholarships are to assist mature women, 25 years of age or older, who are seeking the education necessary for entry into/or advancement within a career in health care. Scholarships are awarded for one year for tuition, fees, and school-related expenses, including child care and transportation. Applications must be postmarked on or before April 15. The maximum award is $1,000. Approximately 50 scholarships are awarded annually. For more information, submit a #10 business-size, self-addressed, double-stamped envelope to: Business and Professional Women's Foundation, Scholarships and Loans, 2012 Massachusetts Avenue, NW, Washington, DC 20036.

NURSES' EDUCATIONAL FUNDS, INC.

5, 8

Nurses' Educational Funds, Inc., sponsors two scholarships for African-American RNs. Awards range from $2,500 to $10,000 each year. The **Estelle Massey Osborne Memorial Scholarship** is for African-American RNs pursuing a master's degree full tim NLN-accredited nursing program. Applicants mu~+ ' (or have declared official intention of becoming bers of a national nursing organization.

The **M. Elizabeth Carnegie Scholarship** African-American RN who is pursuing doctoral stu nursing-related field and demonstrates potential for leadership in the nursing community.

Scholarship kits are $5 to cover the cost of postage and handling. Each scholarship application requires GRE or MAT scores. Deadline for mailing application is February 1. For more information, write: Nurses' Educational Funds, Inc., 555 West 57th Street, New York, NY 10019.

ONCOLOGY NURSING FOUNDATION   3, 4, 5, 6, 7, 8

The Oncology Nursing Foundation offers two (2) scholarships for ethnic minorities. The **Ethnic Minority Bachelor** scholarships award three (3) $2,000 grants to students pursuing a bachelor's degree within the context of their cancer nursing studies. The **Ethnic Minority Master** scholarships award two (2) $3,000 grants to students pursuing a master's degree within the context of their cancer nursing studies. For more information on these scholarship programs, write: Oncology Nursing Foundation, 501 Holiday Drive, Pittsburgh, PA 15220-2749.

PROGRAMS OF EXCELLENCE IN HEALTH   8
PROFESSIONS EDUCATION FOR MINORITIES
PROJECT GRANTS

Grants are awarded to strengthen the national capacity to train minority students in the health professions and to support health professions schools that have trained a significant number of the nation's minority health professionals and enable those schools to supply health professionals to serve minority populations in underserved areas. Grant funds may be used by health professions schools to enhance the academic performance of students in such schools; establish, strengthen, or expand programs to increase the number and quality of applicants for admission to such schools; improve the capacity of the schools to train, recruit, and retain minority faculty; carry out activities to improve the information resources and curricula of the schools and clinical education at the schools, with respect minority issues; and facilitate faculty and student research on health issues particularly affecting minority groups. Funds are available for up to three years, renewable for three-year periods. Deadline dates are announced in the Federal Register.

For further information, please contact: Dr. A. Roland Garcia, Chief, Centers of Excellence Section, Division of Disadvantaged Assistance or John Westcott, Grants Management Officer, Department of Health and Human Services, 5600 Fishers Ln., Parklawn Bldg., Rockville, MD 20857. Telephone (301) 443-4493 or (301) 443-6857.

SWITZER SCHOLARSHIPS FOR WOMEN   8

The Switzer Foundation is a private, nonprofit charitable organization founded in New York City in 1909, under the laws of the State of New York. Members are volunteers selected for their interest and ability to help foundation aims. Switzer Scholarships support training in health service careers and health institutions in the greater New York area. Scholarships are not offered to individuals. Grants are made to educational institutions which then nominate students. For more information, please write to: Switzer Foundation, 350 Hudson Street, New York, NY 10014. Telephone (212) 989-9393, ext. 167.

UNITED NEGRO COLLEGE FUND   1, 3, 8

Scholarships for undergraduate students are awarded through colleges participating in the United Negro College Fund. Awards range from $500 to $7,500. Eight of the participating schools have baccalaureate nursing programs. A list of participating schools may be obtained from: The College Fund/UNCF Program Services, 8260 Willow Oaks Corporate Drive, Fairfax, VA 22031, (800) 331-2244. Requests for information on UNCF scholarships should be directed to the financial aid officer at the schools.

For key to codes showing categories of aid, see page 17.

U.S. PUBLIC HEALTH SERVICE LOAN   1, 3, 4, 5, 8
REPAYMENT PROGRAM
INDIAN HEALTH SERVICE
NATIONAL HEALTH SERVICE CORPS

In 1988, Congress authorized two loan repayment programs for nurses and physicians—one with the **Indian Health Service,** the other with the **National Health Service Corps.** These programs provide total loan repayments directly to lending institutions in exchange for federal and/or private employment commitments. All outstanding health professions education loans, both federal and commercial, apply. The length of commitment is determined by the amount of the loan to be repaid.

For the **Indian Health Service,** nurses must commit to a minimum 2-year service obligation. Loans are repaid up to $30,000 per year. Site visits to Indian Health Service offices prior to final agreement may be offered; most locations are rural. Specialties needed include MSN Nurse Practitioner, Nurse Midwife, Nurse Anesthetist, as well as clinical RNs.

For the **National Health Service Corps,** Primary Care Nurse Practitioners and Certified Nurse-Midwives must commit to a minimum 2-year service obligation. Undergraduate and graduate loans are repaid up to $25,000 per year for first and second years and up to $35,000 for each additional year. Site visits to National Health Service Corps offices prior to final agreement are offered; most locations are rural.

For more information, contact: Loan Repayment Program, Indian Health Service, 12300 Twinbrook Parkway, Suite 100, Rockville, MD 20852. Telephone (301) 443-3396; Loan Repayment Program, National Health Service Corps, 4350 East-West Highway, 10th Floor, Rockville, MD 20857. Telephone (800) 435-6464 or (301) 594-4400.

WILLIAM RANDOLPH HEARST FOUNDATIONS   3, 8

The Hearst Foundation provides grants to programs that aid poverty-level minority groups, educational programs with emphasis on higher education, health delivery systems, and other cultural programs. Note that grants are not provided to individuals. For more information, write: William Randolph Hearst Foundations, 888 Seventh Avenue, 45th Floor, New York, NY 10106-0057.

WOMEN OF THE EVANGELICAL LUTHERAN CHURCH IN AMERICA   3, 5, 8

The Women of the ELCA offers several scholarships to advance nursing education. The maximum amount awarded to any recipient in any one year is $2,000. General criteria includes: applicant must be a laywoman who is also a member of an ELCA congregation; applicant must have experienced an interruption of at least two years in their education since high school; applicant must demonstrate high academic potential and realistic goals; applicant must demonstrate financial need; and applicant must not be preparing for a vocation in the church. For more information and an application, contact: Women of the Evangelical Lutheran Church in America, 8765 West Higgins Road, Chicago, IL 60631. Telephone (312) 380-2730.

WYETH-AYERST LABORATORIES SCHOLARSHIP   7, 8
FOR WOMEN IN GRADUATE MEDICAL AND
HEALTH BUSINESS PROGRAMS

Established in 1993 to assist women in gaining entry into underrepresented and underutilized health-related occupations, particularly in the medical and health business professions, Wyeth-Ayerst offers a **Scholarship for Women in Graduate Medical and Health Business Programs.** The scholarship program encourages women to enter emerging health fields such as biomedical engineering, biomedical research, medical technology, pharmaceutical marketing, public health, and public health policy. This scholarship program, administered by the Business and Professional Women's Foundation Educational Programs through a grant from Wyeth-Ayerst Laboratories, provides $50,000 annually in scholarship grants. Scholarship grants of $2,000 each are awarded for full-time programs of study only at the graduate level. For more information, submit a #10 business-size, self-addressed, double-stamped envelop to: Scholarships and Loans, Business and Professional Women's Foundation, 2012 Massachusetts Avenue, NW, Washington, DC 20036.

Special Awards, Postdoctoral Study, and Research Grants

The aid listed in this chapter is mainly for nurses pursuing studies at or beyond the doctoral level or outside a formal academic course of study. The awards described here also consist largely of grants, traineeships, and fellowships for postdoctoral study, for advanced nursing research, or for other special projects. Other special awards not tied directly to academic study or specifically to nursing are also listed here, so don't overlook this chapter in checking out possible sources of funds.

AGENCY FOR HEALTH CARE POLICY   5, 6, 7
AND RESEARCH
PUBLIC HEALTH SERVICE

The AHCPR offers research grants to doctoral students investigating health care issues in conjunction with their dissertation. The grant provides support up to $30,000 in total direct costs. Grant support is designed to aid the career development of new health service researchers and to encourage the study of complex health service delivery problems. To apply, applicants must be enrolled in an accredited doctoral program in health, medical, social, or management sciences. Proposed studies must be in the areas identified in section 902 of the Public Health Service Act, including: effectiveness, efficiency, and quality of health care services; outcomes of health care services and procedures; clinical practice including primary care and practice-oriented research; health care technologies, facilities, and equipment; health care costs, productivity, and market forces; health promotion and disease prevention; health statistics and epidemiology; and medical liability. This agency also provides individual postdoctoral **National Research Service Awards** related to the organization, financing, and delivery of health services. Priority is given to research projects in primary health promotion and disease prevention, technology assessment, the role of market forces in health care delivery, and studies relevant to issues faced by state and local governments. Current stipends range from $20,000 to $32,000 annually, depending on experience. For more information and an application, write: Director, Office of Scientific Affairs, Executive Office Center, 2101 E. Jefferson Street, Suite 400, Rockville, MD 20852. Telephone (301) 594-1449.

AMERICAN ASSOCIATION OF CRITICAL-CARE   4, 5
NURSES NELLCOR-AACN MENTORSHIP GRANT

The **Nellcor-AACNMentorship Grant** facilitates critical-care nursing practice research between a novice and an experienced researcher. The novice researcher must be a beginning researcher with limited or no research experience in the area of the proposed investigation, have RN licensure, be a member of AACN, and may use the grant to fund research for an academic degree. The mentor must show strong evidence of research in the area of the proposed investigation and must not be conducting such research as part of an academic degree. The novice investigator can receive up to $10,000 per grant award. The deadline for proposals is February 1. For more information contact: Grants Administrator, American Association of Critical-Care Nurses, 101 Columbia, Aliso Viejo, CA 92656-1491.

AMERICAN ASSOCIATION OF   3, 4, 7
OCCUPATIONAL HEALTH NURSES, INC. (AAOHN)

In the area of occupational health nursing practice, AAOHN sponsors three annual research awards open to nursing students and clinical practitioners who are contributing to the occupational health nursing knowledge base: **Mary Louise Brown Research Award**

($3,000), **Otis Clapp Research Award** ($2,000), and **American Board of Occupational Health Nurses** ($1,000). AAOHN also provides one annual academic scholarship, the **Charles J. Turcott Academic Scholarship Award** ($2,000), open only to AAOHN members currently enrolled in baccalaureate, masters, or doctoral nursing programs. To obtain more information on these AAOHN awards, write to: AAOHN Awards, AAOHN, 50 Lenox Pointe, Atlanta, GA 30324-3176. Telephone (404) 262-1162.

AMERICAN ASSOCIATION OF UNIVERSITY WOMEN EDUCATIONAL FOUNDATION   7

The Association grants fellowships to reward women who have achieved distinction or the promise of distinction in their respective fields, including nursing. Importance is attached to the individual project proposed on the application. Women are eligible who have (1) outstanding scholarly achievement and (2) are engaged in dissertation or postdoctoral research. Fellowship awards are currently $13,000 to $15,000 for dissertation research and $20,000 to $25,000 for postdoctoral research for one year of study beginning in July. The application deadline is November of each year. For more information and an application, contact: American Association of University Women Educational Foundation, 1111 16th Street, NW, Washington, DC 20036. Telephone (202) 728-7603.

AMERICAN LUNG ASSOCIATION   6, 7

The American Lung Association's **Research Training Fellowships** are available to holders of doctoral degrees who are interested in further training as scientific investigators in the field of prevention and control of lung disease. Applicants are expected to have obtained an appointment in a university, medical center, or hospital for training under a responsible teacher or investigator. Preference will be given to applicants whose program of training will enable them to pursue an academic career. Candidates must demonstrate the relevance and value of their proposed training to the understanding and treatment of lung disease. Support will not be awarded beyond the third postdoctoral year.

For key to codes showing categories of aid, see page 17.

Awards are made on an annual basis for amounts of up to $32,500 the first year and $32,500 for a second year. The application deadline is October 1, and decisions are made in late January.

The **Lung Health Research Dissertation Grant** provides support for doctoral research training to individuals conducting dissertation research on issues relevant to people with lung disease. The grant is for students from various disciplines of the behavioral and social sciences. Nurses pursuing a doctoral degree in any field are eligible. You must be a United States Citizen, a Canadian Citizen, or permanent resident of the U.S. enrolled in a U.S. institution. This grant is for two years at $21,000 per year. This grant may also be used for stipend and research support.

Application forms may be obtained from: American Lung Association, Medical Affairs Division, 1740 Broadway, New York, NY 10019-4374.

AMERICAN NEPHROLOGY NURSES'   3, 4, 7
ASSOCIATION

The American Nephrology Nurses' Association has many awards and fellowships available to ANNA members for nephrology research. The application deadline is November of each year, and recipients are notified in February or March. For application forms and information on these and other grants and awards available to ANNA members, contact: Chairperson, Awards Committee, East Holly Avenue, Box 56, Pitman, NJ 08071-0056. Telephone (609) 256-2320.

AMERICAN NURSES FOUNDATION, NURSING   4, 5, 7
RESEARCH GRANTS PROGRAM

The American Nurses Foundation offers the **Nursing Research Grant** for beginning and advanced nursing researchers. The awards range from $2,500–$10,000 for a one-year research project conducted by a registered nurse. For more information, contact: American Nurses Foundation, Nursing Research Grant, 600 Maryland Avenue, SW, Suite 100W, Washington, DC 20024. Telephone (202) 651-7298, WWW http://www.nursingworld.org/anf/anf@ana.org Subject: NRG.

AMERICAN SOCIETY FOR PARENTERAL AND 4, 7
ENTERAL NUTRITION RESEARCH GRANTS

Grants offered fund research in nutrition support and clinical nutrition by new or young investigators. Applicants from the nursing, medical, dietetic, and pharmaceutical professions are encouraged. One award up to $25,000 per year and two awards up $5,000 per year are offered. Applications are due October 13 of the preceding year in which the award takes place. For further information and applications forms, contact: Director, American Society for Parenteral and Enteral Nutrition, Research Grants, 8630 Fenton St., Ste. 412, Silver Springs, MD 20910.

ARTHRITIS FOUNDATION 5, 6, 7

The Arthritis Foundation currently offers three grants. The **New Investigator Grant for Arthritis Health Professionals** is given to design and carry out innovative research projects related to rheumatic diseases. Applicants need not be associated with an arthritis unit, but must have demonstrated interest in rheumatology practice, research, or education. Suitable areas include, but are not limited to, functional behavioral, nutritional, occupational, or epidemiological aspects of patient care and management. Grants are awarded to both new and experienced investigators. Applicants who have received a doctoral degree within the last five years are particularly encouraged. Awards are made for up to two years, usually in the amount of $25,000 per year, and may be renewable for a third year. Grantees are expected to submit regular reports and publish the results. Candidates must have a doctoral degree or equivalent, demonstrated research experience, or a supervisor or coinvestigator with demonstrated research experience in the area of study, and membership or eligibility for membership in their national professional organization. Projects are judged on design, originality, potential significance, relevance to rheumatic diseases, and researcher's background and experience.

The **Doctoral Dissertation Award for Arthritis Health Professionals** is given to advance the research training of arthritis health professionals in investigative or clinical teaching careers as they relate to rheumatic diseases. Grants are awarded to doctoral candidates entering the research phase of their programs, with stipends up to $10,000 per year, and to be considered as salary or research expenses.

For key to codes showing categories of aid, see page 17.

Suitable studies include, but are not limited to, functional behavioral, nutritional, occupational, or epidemiological aspects of patient care and management. Candidates must have membership or eligibility for membership in their professional organization.

The **Clinical Science Grants** encourage and support original research on problems related to the diagnosis, prognosis, and management of adults and children with arthritis and rheumatic diseases. Individuals with doctoral degrees (PhD, DO, MD or equivalent) at the assistant professor level or higher at any nonprofit institution in the U.S. are eligible to apply. Grants are made up to five years for $80,000 per year.

For these awards, applications are available May 1, with a submission deadline of September 1. For further information contact: The Arthritis Foundation, Dodie M. Porter, Research Department, 1330 West Peachtree Street, Atlanta, GA 30309. Telephone (404) 872-7100, ext. 6311, fax (404) 877-3170, e-mail dporter@arthritis .org, WWW http://www.arthritis.org.

ASSOCIATION OF UNIVERSITY PROGRAMS   7
IN HEALTH ADMINISTRATION
(INVESTING IN THE FUTURE OF HEALTH
MANAGEMENT LEADERS)

The Association of University Programs in Health Administration (AUPHA), the preeminent international consortium of educational centers for health care services management and policy, was founded 46 years ago with support from the W.K. Kellogg Foundation. It is the only non-profit entity of its kind worldwide whose mission is to improve health status and the quality of health care services by strengthening the capacity to educate health services managers.

AUPHA is an operating consortium whose membership includes 105 university programs in North America and 60 affiliated training centers in 32 countries around the world. Its resources include 250 directly affiliated hospitals and health centers, 600 individual members and many corporations and organizations committed to its mission. AUPHA draws extensively upon these members who have agreed to make their resources available to AUPHA for consultative purposes. In addition, they are available for use as training sites for visiting health care management executives, academics, trainers and policy makers.

In each country in which it works, AUPHA commits resources to help universities, other training institutions, ministries of health and practicing executives develop the management expertise and related resources to improve health status through excellence in education and training technologies. AUPHA maintains a continuing support system so affiliated training programs in healthcare management and policy will not operate in isolation or without a permanent technical support system through private and public funding.

The following award is offered by the AUPHA: **The Baxter Foundation Prize** is administered by the Association of University Programs in Health Administration (AUPHA). The prize recognizes an unusually significant contribution to improved public medical care through innovative health services research. An individual's specific contribution or a career-long achievement may be recognized.

The Baxter Foundation Prize for distinction in health services is awarded to an individual working in any relevant discipline, anywhere in the world. To ensure that prize recipients represent leaders in and major contributors to health services research internationally, nominations are actively solicited.

Nominations must provide complete documentation including: a statement of accomplishments that distinguishes the nominee's contributions from the work of others, evidence of impact through publications and testimonials of leaders, copies of relevant publications, and a resume. Letters of support are also invited. One letter of nomination and two letters of recommendation are *required*.

The prize consists of an individual award of $10,000. In addition, $15,000 will be awarded to the institution designated by the recipient to support his or her work. The prize focuses on: Health Services Management, Health Policy Development, and Healthcare Delivery.

All materials must be received by February 1 of each year to be considered for that year's prize. Nominations should be in English. Supporting materials may be in other languages.

For more information, contact: the Secretary, HSR Prize Committee, AUPHA, 1911 North Fort Myer Drive, Suite 503, Arlington, VA 22209. Telephone (703) 524-5500.

BAXTER ALLEGIANCE FOUNDATION GRANT   7, 8

The Baxter Allegiance Foundation offers grants for programs that improve quality and cost-effectiveness in health care delivery systems and increases access to care. The foundation also supports programs that work to improve career prospects in health care for minorities, women, and the disabled. The Baxter Allegiance Foundation accepts grant proposals throughout the year. For further information on Foundation Grant awards, contact: Executive Director, Baxter Allegiance Foundation, One Baxter Parkway, Deerfield, IL 60015.

BUREAU OF HEALTH PROFESSIONS   7
DIVISION OF NURSING
U.S. DEPARTMENT OF HEALTH AND HUMAN SERVICES

Special Projects Grants and Contracts are authorized under the Public Health Service Act to improve nursing practice through projects that increase the knowledge and skills of nursing personnel, enhance their effectiveness in primary health care delivery, and increase the number of qualified professional nurses.

Grants and contracts may be awarded to public and nonprofit private entities that meet at least one of the following criteria: (a) increases the number of students enrolled in programs of professional nursing, (b) establishes or expands nursing practice arrangements in noninstitutional settings to demonstrate methods to improve access to primary health care in medically underserved areas, (c) provides continuing education for nurses serving in medically underserved communities, and (d) provides fellowships to individuals who are employed by nursing facilities or home health agencies as nursing paraprofessionals.

Information concerning all programs can be obtained from the Internet and the Bureau's Bulletin Board. All competitive grant problems are announced in the Federal Register. Inquiries regarding grants management should be addressed to: Grants Management Officer (D-10), Bureau of Health Professions, Parklawn Building, Room 8C-26, 5600 Fishers Ln., Rockville, MD 20857. Telephone (310) 443-6333.

CANADIAN NURSES FOUNDATION   7
STUDY AWARDS AND RESEARCH GRANTS

Grants provide funding for nurses undertaking university studies in nursing and health care and for research related to nursing practice and health care. Study awards are given for university study at the baccalaureate, master's, and doctoral levels. Priority will be given to nurses studying in programs with a nursing focus. Once recipients have completed their degrees, they must return to nursing and assist in the development of improved nursing and health care in Canada. Applications for study awards must be received by April 15th and June 15th for research grants. For further information, contact: Beverly Campbell, Executive Director, Canadian Nurses Foundation, 50 Driveway, Ottawa ON K2P 1E2, Canada. Telephone (613) 237-2133, WWW http://www.magma.ca/~cnf.

CANADIAN NURSES RESPIRATORY SOCIETY   5, 6, 7

CNRS offers fellowships and research grants. Fellowships are offered to registered nurses pursuing postgraduate education with a major component of the program involving respiratory nursing practice. Grants for research and feasibility studies are offered to registered nurses undertaking research investigations related to nursing management of patients with respiratory disease and symptoms.

For fellowships, an applicant must be a Canadian citizen or a permanent Canadian resident, be a Registered Nurse, be enrolled or accepted for full-time studies in a graduate program at the masters or doctorate level, and be a member of CNRS.

For research grants, the principal investigator must be a Canadian citizen or a permanent Canadian resident, be a Registered Nurse, hold an appointment in, or have an affiliation with, a health care agency, education institution, or other organization in Canada that can administer the funds in an approved manner, and be a member of CNRS.

Financial support per award: *Fellowship:* $2,000 to $8,000; *Research Grants:* $3,000 to $30,000. Deadline is November 1, 1997. Duration of the support is one year.

For more information and applications, write: The Lung Association, 1900 City Park Drive, Suite 508, Gloucester, ON K1J 1A3,

For key to codes showing categories of aid, see page 17.

Canada. Telephone (613) 747-6776, fax (613) 747-7430, WWW, http://www.lung.ca.

COUNCIL FOR RESEARCH IN   **4, 7**
NURSING EDUCATION
CALLS FOR GRANT PROPOSALS

The National League for Nursing Council for Research in Nursing Education (NLN-CRNE) is sponsoring small grant awards for research in nursing education. One to three awards ranging from $5,000 to $10,000 will be given for nursing education research. Priority will be given to applications that reflect outcomes of: community-focused education; innovative educational models; changes in the teaching and learning environments; and collaboration with other disciplines in use of technology in nursing education and nursing education research. Principal investigators must be individual members of the Council for Research in Nursing Education. The proposal will be evaluated on the following criteria: purpose of study, theoretical basis, significance; methods, including proposed analysis; feasibility; protection of human subjects; time line; a budget that demonstrates feasibility; and documented ability to conduct the study.

Project length should not exceed two years. All projects will require one mid-point progress report and a final report. Reports will be presented by researchers at the CRNE meeting following completion of the project. Applicants must submit eight (8) copies of the proposal, postmarked by May 1, 1998, to: Lynda Crawford, PhD, RN, Associate Director of Community Health Research, National League for Nursing, 350 Hudson Street, New York, NY 10014.

ENVIRONMENTAL HEALTH AND NURSING   **7**
SCIENCES NRSAs

NIEHS and NINR are interested in receiving individual and institutional National Research Service Award applications for support of training at the pre- and postdoctoral level of nurses interested in pursuing research careers combining environmental health and nursing sciences. The purpose is to provide a cadre of nurse investigators who are prepared to apply the principles of clinical nursing research to environmental research problems. Prospective applicants will need to contact program officers for specific eligibility requirements and application deadline.

For further information, please contact: Dr. Allen Dearry, Chemical Exposure and Molecular Biology Branch, (919) 541-4943; e-mail: dearry@niehs.nih.gov; Dr. Michael Galvin, Organ and Systems Toxicology Branch, (919) 541-7825; e-mail galvin@niehs.nih.gov; David Mineo, Chief, Grants Management Officer, (919) 541-7628; e-mail mineo@niehs.nih.gov; at the National Institute of Environmental Health Sciences, PO Box 12233, Research Triangle Park, NC 27709.

EPILEPSY FOUNDATION OF AMERICA 7

The Epilepsy Foundation of America offers research grants and research training fellowships. One-year research grants are awarded to support basic and clinical research in the biological, behavioral and social sciences which will advance the understanding, treatment and prevention of epilepsy. Priority is given to beginning investigators just entering the field of epilepsy research, to new or innovative projects, and to investigators whose research is relevant to developmental or pediatric aspects of epilepsy. Applications in the behavioral sciences are encouraged.

Applications from established investigators with other sources of support are discouraged. Research grants are not intended to provide support for postdoctoral fellows. Support is limited to $30,000.

Research training fellowships offer qualified individuals the opportunity to develop expertise in epilepsy research through a one-year training experience and involvement in an epilepsy research project. The research project may be either basic or clinical but must address a question of fundamental importance. A clinical training component is not required. Preference is given to applicants whose proposals have a pediatric or developmental emphasis.

The Fellowships carry a $30,000 stipend and must be carried out at a facility where there is an ongoing epilepsy research program. For more information and applications, write: Epilepsy Foundation of America, Postdoctoral Fellowships/Research Grants in Behavioral Sciences, 4351 Garden City Drive, Suite 406, Landover, MD 20785.

FIRST INDEPENDENT RESEARCH   5, 7
SUPPORT AND TRANSITION (FIRST) AWARDS

FIRST awards support small studies of high quality carried out by new investigators to help them develop their research capabilities and demonstrate the merit of their research. FIRST awards provide funds for five years. Only domestic organizations and institutions are eligible to receive FIRST awards. As recipient, the principal investigator must be a beginning investigator who does not hold training status at the time the award begins. Application deadlines are February 1, June 1, and October 1. For applications and guidelines contact: Office of Grant Information, Extramural Outreach and Information Resources, Office of Extramural Research, National Institutes of Health, 6701 Rockledge Drive, Suite 6095, Bethesda, MD 20892. Telephone (301) 435-0714, fax (301) 480-0525, e-mail asknih@odrockm1.od.nih.gov, WWW http://www.nih.gov.

GERIATRIC MENTAL HEALTH ACADEMIC AWARDS   5, 7

This award is to assist in the development of academically situated, research-oriented persons in the area of mental disorders of the aging. The award, made to an institution, provides a faculty member who is a psychiatrist, psychiatric nurse, psychologist, or social worker with the opportunity of five years of study and supervised experience to prepare for a faculty leadership role in geriatric mental health research. Applications are encouraged from women and minority faculty, as well as from historically minority institutions. Salary support is provided. Applicants must have advanced degrees in one of the core health disciplines. The amount of the award is for salary (up to $75,000), and research/training activities (up $50,000). Applications are due February 1, June 1, or October 1. For more information and an application, write: Enid Light, PhD, Mental Disorders of the Aging Research Branch, Division of Clinical Research, Rm. 18-101. Telephone (301) 443-1185; or Bruce Ringler, Grants Management Officer, National Institutes of Health, 5600 Fishers Lane, Parklawn Building, Rockville, MD 20587.

HEALTH CANADA'S NATIONAL HEALTH RESEARCH AND DEVELOPMENT PROGRAM (NHRDP) CAREER AWARDS PROGRAM   7

Postdoctoral Fellowships are offered to highly qualified candidates who have completed all formal academic training and who wish to acquire up to two years supervised research experience in population health or health care in an established health research setting. Fellowships are only tenable in Canadian centers. To be eligible, candidates must hold a PhD (or equivalent research doctorate) in a research field closely associated with public health or health services, or an MD/ DDS, and a Master's degree in an appropriate health research field.

The **National Health Research Scholar** award is intended to afford exceptionally promising investigators with proven research abilities the freedom to pursue population-health research relevant to NHRDP missions on a full-time basis for a period of up to five years. To be eligible, candidates must possess the same academic qualifications required of Postdoctoral Fellows. In addition, they must provide evidence of having had not less than two and not more than six years of proven research experience in population-health enquiry after completing their highest research degree. Without exception, awards are tenable only in Canada.

The **National Health Scientist Award** is designed to foster a high level of health research activity in Canada by providing acknowledged leaders in population-health enquiry the opportunity to pursue a full-time research career. To be eligible, candidates must possess the same academic qualifications required of Postdoctoral Fellows and must have demonstrated outstanding competence in and commitment to population-based health research for a minimum of ten years following completion of all formal academic training. Without exception, awards are tenable only in Canada.

For more information, please contact: Information Officer, Research and Program Policy Directorate, Health Promotion and Programs Branch, Health Canada, Ottawa, Ontario, K1A 1B4, Canada. Postal Locator: 1912. Telephone (613) 954-8549, fax (613) 954-7363.

For key to codes showing categories of aid, see page 17.

HEART AND STROKE FOUNDATION   4, 5, 7
OF ONTARIO STROKE
INVESTIGATOR AWARD

This award is given to develop and enhance stroke research in Ontario, Canada. For the fiscal year 1997/1998, two entry-level (fellowship equivalent) awards will be offered to qualified candidates who have completed all formal academic training and who wish to acquire two to three years of supervised research experience in an established research setting, working with an identified academic supervisor. The award is intended for applicants with an MD, PhD, or equivalent degree. Applicants must have a strong interest in pursuing a career in stroke research.

The Foundation expects nominating institutions to offer successful candidates a full-time faculty, staff, or equivalent position, with no less than 75 percent effort reserved for research, subject to satisfactory performance in the research training period. This commitment is required at the time of the initial application and with request for the renewal of support.

Upon completion of the first term of the award (two to three years), investigators who have successfully completed their training may apply for a second three-year term of fellowship-level support (Phase Two). Along with the salary contribution, Phase Two provides an annual supplement for essential equipment and/or supplies.

Phase Three of the Stroke Investigator Award consists of five years of salary support at the scholarship level. Stroke investigators who have not completed Phase One and Two, but who meet the requirements for a Heart and Stroke Foundation Scholarship may apply. Applications must be submitted by the sponsoring institution for new, as opposed to existing, faculties. Successful applicants may apply for a second, five-year period of scholarship-level support.

Applications for the first phase of fellowship-level support must be submitted by November 15, for commencement July 1, 1998. Junior personnel (fellowship) application forms may be obtained from the research office of the institution or by contacting the Heart and Stroke Foundation of Canada. For further information, please contact: Miss Evelyn T. McGloin, V.P., Research Administration, Heart and Stroke Foundation of Ontario, 477 Mt. Pleasant Road, 4th Flr., Toronto, Ontario M4S 2L9. Telephone (416) 489-7111, ext. 318; fax (416) 489-9015 or (416) 481-3439.

For key to codes showing categories of aid, see page 17.

HEART AND STROKE FOUNDATIONS OF CANADA NURSING RESEARCH FELLOWSHIPS   5, 7, 8

This fellowship is an in-training award for persons working toward a master's or doctoral degree specializing in cardiovascular or cerebrovascular nursing. For master's degree candidates, the program must include a requirement for a research project or thesis. The fellowship is tenable for a maximum of two years. Applications for work in an academic setting with research content for one year of study within or outside of Canada will be considered. The award is for C$25,000 per year with a C$1,000 per year incentive for travel for scientific purposes. The deadline is March 15. For more information and an application, write: Heart and Stroke Foundation of Canada Nursing Research Fellowships, Division of Research Administration, Heart and Stroke Foundation of Canada, 160 George Street, Suite 200, Ottawa, ON K1N 9M2. WWW http://www.hsf.ca/research/

INTERNATIONAL ASSOCIATION OF GERONTOLOGY   4, 7

The International Association of Gerontology's **Sandoz Prize for Gerontological Research** is available to individuals and groups directly engaged in research in some area of gerontology or geriatrics. Candidates can be nominated by third parties. The value of the prize is worth a total of Sfr. 20,000.

Awards are made every two years with the next to be presented in June of 1997. For application deadlines and more information, write to: Manfred Bergener, MD, Liaison Officer IAG for the Sandoz Prize for Gerontological Research, Rheinishe Landesklinik, Wilhelm-Greisinger Strasse 23, D-5000 Koln 91, Federal Republic of Germany. Information can also be obtained from any Sandoz company.

LILLIAN SHOLTIS BRUNNER SUMMER FELLOWSHIP FOR HISTORICAL RESEARCH IN NURSING   5, 7

The **Lillian Sholtis Brunner Summer Fellowship for Historical Research in Nursing** supports six to eight weeks of residential study and use of collections at the Center for the Study of the History of

Nursing. The amount of the fellowship is $2,500. Selection of Brunner Fellows will be based on evidence of preparation and/or productivity in historical research related to nursing. Brunner fellows will work under the general direction of nurse historians associated with the Center. The application deadline for this fellowship is December 31, 1997.

The **Alice Fisher Society Historical Scholarship,** a $2,500 award, is open to nurses at the master or doctoral level who are seeking assistance with research and writing as part of their study of history. Each scholar is expected to spend four to six weeks in residence at the Center. The application deadline for this scholarship is December 31, 1998.

For more information and applications, write: Center Director, The Center for the Study of the History of Nursing, School of Nursing, University of Pennsylvania, 307 Nursing Education Building, Philadelphia, PA 19104-6906. Or e-mail us at history@pobox.upenn.edu or refer to our website: http://www .upenn.edu/nursing/facres_history.html.

MICHIGAN NURSES ASSOCIATION   7

Every two years the Michigan Nurses Association sponsors a competitive award to promote nursing research in Michigan. The Conduct and Utilization of Research in Nursing (CURN) Award funds either for the conduction of research or utilization of studies that have a direct impact on patient care. The recipient receives $2,000. Proposals for the 1997 CURN Scholar Award are due July 1. For more information, contact: Jan Coye, Michigan Nurses Association, 2310 Jolly Oak Road, Okemos, MI 48864. Telephone (517) 349-5640.

NATIONAL CANCER INSTITUTE CANCER   7
PREVENTION AND CONTROL RESEARCH
SMALL GRANTS PROGRAMS

New and experienced investigators in nursing and other relevant fields and disciplines may apply for small grants to test ideas or do pilot studies. Cancer control program areas appropriate for research grants include human intervention research in the following areas; prevention; pilot studies of new methods of screening and early detection; cancer control sciences studies to change current behaviors and/or institute new behaviors or health promotion interventions effective in reducing incidence, morbidity, or mortality from cancer; and smoking prevention and cessation pilot studies targeted at improving utilization of current technologies in target populations or organizations. Additional areas of interest are applications research in modifying, feasibility testing, and adopting proven state-of-the-art intervention programs and strategies from other research projects for use in special populations, state and local health agencies, or other studies aimed at developing cancer control interventions, or cancer control operations research and evaluation studies; community oncology (improving into community settings); and applied epidemiology (using epidemiologic methods to determine the association between exposure to an intervention and its impact on disease). Additional information may be obtained electronically through the NIH grant line (301) 402-2221 and the NIH gopher (gopher.nih.gov) and by mail and e-mail. Investigators who are interested in conducting exploratory studies in cancer control research and who have never received NCI cancer control funding are eligible to apply. This includes students enrolled in an accredited doctoral degree program. For further information, contact: Helen Meissner, Division of Cancer Prevention and Control, National Cancer Institute, 6130 Executive Blvd, Executive Plaza N., Bethesda, MD 20892. Telephone (301) 496-8520, e-mail meissenh@dcpceps.nci.nih.gov.

NATIONAL CANCER INSTITUTE   5, 6
NATIONAL RESEARCH SERVICE AWARD
INDIVIDUAL PREDOCTORAL RESEARCH
FELLOWSHIP FOR ONCOLOGY NURSES

The National Cancer Institute (NCI) in collaboration with the National Center for Nursing Research announces the availability of a limited number of **National Research Service Predoctoral Fellowship Awards for Oncology Nurses.** This program is intended to encourage selected oncology nurses to prepare for academic research careers. The award will enable trainees in pursuit of a PhD degree in basic or applied cancer science to undertake up to five years of special study and supervised research experience tailored to individual needs.

Applicants must be citizens of the United States or its possessions and territories, or must have been lawfully admitted to the United States and hold a I-151 or I-551 card. Applicants must possess at least a bachelor's degree in nursing and a current registered nurse license. Applicants also must have been accepted for training at the postbaccalaureate level in a program designed to culminate in a doctorate. Applicants in programs leading only to a master's degree will not qualify. Applicants must have one or more sponsors or advisors who are recognized as accomplished investigators in the discipline. Awardees and sponsors will be required to submit a progress report at the end of each year of support. For more information and an application, contact: Program Director, Cancer Training Branch, CTP, DCTDC, EPN520, National Cancer Institute, Bethesda, MD 20892. Telephone (301) 496-8580.

NATIONAL FOUNDATION FOR INFECTIOUS   4, 5, 7
DISEASES YOUNG INVESTIGATOR
MATCHING GRANTS

The National Foundation for Infectious Diseases Young Investigator Matching Grants are intended to assist young investigators who are beginning their research. Each application must be accompanied by an agreement from the applicant's sponsoring institution to match the $2,000 award with equal funds. Each young investigator must be a legal resident or citizen of the United States or Canada with full-time junior faculty (instructor or assistant professor) status at a recognized and accredited institution of higher learning in the United States or Canada. Priority will be given to those who do not have research grants and whose studies represent pilot work with an intent to further develop their research. Grant proposals must be based on research relevant to infectious diseases, microbiology, clinical medicine, epidemiology, nursing, etc. Those topics included in the "top ten" infectious diseases problems as recognized by the NFID will receive highest priority for funding, as follows: HIV and AIDS; Antimicrobial Resistance and Emerging Infections; Vaccine Preventable Diseases (including flu); Hospital Acquired and Opportunistic Infections; Viral Hepatitis, Gastrointestinal, Diarrheal and

Foodborne Diseases; Sexually Transmitted Diseases; Tuberculosis; Zoonotic Diseases; and Tropical Infectious Diseases.

Application forms are available upon request from the National Foundation for Infectious Diseases. Address applications to: NFID, 4733 Bethesda Avenue, Suite 750, Bethesda, MD 20814. Applications should be postmarked no later than February 15.

NATIONAL HEART, LUNG, AND BLOOD INSTITUTE   8
MINORITY SHORT-TERM TRAINING GRANTS

These grants support short-term research training experience of two to three months duration for minority undergraduate students, minority students in health professional schools, and minority graduate students. The program objectives are to bolster the exposure of minority students to opportunities inherent in research careers in the areas relevant to cardiovascular, pulmonary, and hematologic diseases and to bolster the already short supply of minority investigators by attracting highly qualified minority students into biomedical and behavioral research careers. Trainees appointed to the program need not be from the grantee institution but may include a number of minority students from other institutions. Institutions may request up to five years of support for at least four and not more than 24 trainees per year. For further information contact: Mary Reilly, Division of Lung Diseases, National Heart, Lung, and Blood Institute, 6701 Rockledge Dr. MSC 7952, Bethesda, MD 20892. Telephone (301) 435-0222, fax (301) 480-3557, e-mail maryreilly@nih.gov.

NATIONAL INSTITUTE ON AGING   7

The NIA offers a variety of research grants to nurses and nurse-associated health scientists in diverse subject areas. These grants are usually awarded to institutions for the initiation or expansion of research agendas by individual research scientists. The **Osteoarthritis Research Grants** intend to stimulate research that provides an improved understanding of general and age-specific epidemiology, etiology (including age-related changes in function or metabolism) and prevention and treatment of osteoarthritis. Multidisciplinary research approaches are emphasized. Investigators interested in this program are invited to write or call NIA program staff prior to submission of a formal proposal.

The **Cognitive Aging Processes Research Grants** supports research and research training on age-related constancy and change in basic cognitive mechanisms including learning, memory, attention, language, concept formation, and differentiation of abnormal from normal processes.

The **Behavior Change and Prevention Strategies to Reduce Transmission of AIDS Research Grants** supports research to identify ways to change behaviors that place persons at high risk for AIDS infection. Applicants may request support for up to five years. Support is available for a traditional research project, small grant, FIRST award, program project award, independent scientist award, mentored clinical scientist development award, or research center grant.

The **Alzheimer's Disease Etiology Research Grants** promote investigations on the etiology or pathogenesis of Alzheimer's disease, including studies of the role of genetics, immune function, endocrine function, nutrition, stress, trauma, toxins, infections, and more.

The **Health and Effective Functioning in the Middle and Later Years Research Grants** support research to specify how psychological processes, interacting with biological processes, influence health and functioning in the middle and later years. Appropriate research topics have included work and retirement, health institutions, social support, health behaviors and attitudes, personality, nutrition, exercise, sleep, family and household, and methodological studies. Written and telephone inquires are encouraged.

The **Teaching Nursing Home Program Awards** support research by academic centers and nursing homes on health problems, therapies, and health maintenance strategies for older persons in nursing homes as well as other institutional and community settings. The maximum duration of new awards and of competitive renewals is five years; projects may be extended through competitive renewal applications to a maximum total project period of eight years.

Specific information on the grants noted above may be obtained from Dr. Richard Sprott, Biology of Aging, (301) 496-4996; Dr. Evan Hadley, Geriatrics and Clinical Research, (301) 496-6761; Dr. Neil Buckholtz, Behavioral and Social Research, (301) 496-3136; Dr. Zaven Khachaturian, Neuroscience and Neuropsychology of Aging Research, (301) 496-9350; Dr. Miriam Kelty, Small Business Innovation Research, (301) 496-9322; or Joseph Ellis, Grants Management Officer (301) 496-1472. Or write to: National Institute on Aging, 7201 Wisconsin Avenue, Gateway Bldg., Bethesda, MD 20892.

The **Mentored Research Scientist Development Award** is for research scientists who have established careers in biomedical, behavioral, or social research and wish to change career direction toward aging research; more junior researchers with training in aging research who need an additional period of mentored research experience prior to becoming fully independent; or researchers with training and experience in some aspect of aging research who wish to gain complimentary training to expand their research interests in aging. More information on this grant may be obtained by e-mail or through the NIH grant line (301) 402-2221, the NIH gopher (gopher.nih.gov), and the NIH website (gttp://www.nih.gov).

NATIONAL INSTITUTE OF CHILD HEALTH AND HUMAN DEVELOPMENT BREASTFEEDING AND HUMAN MILK RESEARCH GRANTS   7

The NICHD seeks to support applications dealing with the process of lactation and the biology of human milk. The goals of this research are to understand causal mechanisms and to improve public health. Particular areas of interest include the determinants of breastfeeding in different populations, the nature of the physiological processes involved in milk formation and secretion, and the function of human milk components in infant health. For further information contact: Hildegard Topper, National Institute of Child Health and Human Development, 9000 Rockville Pike, Bldg. 31, Bethesda, MD 20892. Telephone (301) 496-1848.

NATIONAL INSTITUTE OF MENTAL HEALTH   7

The NIMH offers a variety of research grants to nurses and nurse-associated health scientists in diverse subject areas. These grants are usually awarded to institutions for the initiation or expansion of research agendas by individual research scientists. The **Schizophrenia**

Academic Awards assist in the development of academically situated, research-oriented persons in the areas of schizophrenia. The award, made to an institution, provides a faculty member who is a psychiatrist or psychiatric nurse with the opportunity for five years of special study and supervised experience to prepare for a faculty leadership role in schizophrenia research. Salary support is provided. Potential applicants must be psychiatrists or psychiatric nurses with master's degrees. All grant applications are due February 1, June 1, or October 1.

The **Mental Health Services in General Health Care Research Grants** encourage research on the nature, recognition, classification, treatment and outcomes of people with mental disorders in primary care and other general medical/health settings. Applications may be submitted by foreign and domestic, public and private, and nonprofit and for-profit organizations and institutions.

The **Aging Women and Breast Cancer Grants** are sponsored by NIMH via support from the National Cancer Institute, the National Institute on Aging, and the National Institute of Nursing Research. Their purpose is to expand the knowledge base on breast cancer in older women through studies in the fields of biology, clinical medicine, epidemiology, and the behavioral and social sciences. Specific information on this grant may be obtained by two electronic addresses: e-mail Dr. Enid Light. (elight@nih.gov) at the Mental Disorders of the Aging Research Branch or via the NIH website (http://www.nih.gov).

For further information on these and other nursing dedicated grants, contact: Division of Clinical Research, National Institute of Mental Health, 5600 Fishers LN, Parklawn Bldg., Rockville, MD 20857.

NATIONAL INSTITUTE OF NURSING RESEARCH　　　7

The NINR offers a variety of research grants to nurses in diverse subject areas. These grants are awarded either to individual nurse researchers affiliated with recognized institutions for nursing research or to such institutions themselves for disbursement to individual nurse researchers. The **Postdoctoral Training Opportunities for Nurses in NIH Intramural Programs Grants** provide a research environment and supervision of nurses holding the doctorate who wish to spend one to three years in postdoctoral research training. Individuals interested in applying for the fellowship should contact the appropriate laboratory to discuss the research training experiences available.

The **Nursing Research Related to AIDS Grants** is an NINR priority area. Researchers should focus on research designed to enhance AIDS prevention and to improve mechanisms for providing nursing care to acute and long-term AIDS patients. Topics of interest range from the etiology of AIDS patients at various stages of the disease to public policy issues such as methods of early screening and diagnosis/control of the spread of the disease, and integration of patients, including infants and young children, in community settings.

The **Nursing Systems Research Grants** support research on the environment in which nursing care is delivered. Projects that investigate promising approaches to nursing management and nursing care delivery are of special interest. Topics of interest also range from outcomes of home care, long-term care, and/or hospital care to the ethical issues related to patient care and patient care research.

The **Nursing Research Project Grants** are intended to enlarge the body of scientific knowledge that underlies nursing practice, education, and nursing services administration and which has practical effect through utilization of such knowledge.

The **NINR Grants and Training Awards** support basic and clinical research and research training in the science of health care relevant to nursing. The research programs supported address actual and potential health problems, from health promotion and disease prevention to the ethics of patient care.

The **Nursing and Biology Interface Small Grants Program** intends to stimulate nurse investigators to explore innovative, state-of-the-art science research using biological technology. Keys here are the successful outcomes of such research to advance studies linking basic biological sciences with nursing clinical questions and nursing studies having a biological focus, and to facilitate use of state-of-the-art science biological techniques by nurse researchers.

The **Postdoctoral Research Extramural Training Grants** support individuals with an RN who hold an earned doctorate for up to three years of full-time research training in areas of interest to the NINR. In support of studies of nursing interventions, procedures, delivery methods, and ethics of patient care, NINR programs are

For key to codes showing categories of aid, see page 17.

expected to complement other biomedical research programs concerned primarily with causes and treatment of disease.

The **Nursing Research Training Fellowships Related to Alzheimer's Disease and Related Disorder Grants** support research training in areas related to patient care. Qualified pre- and postdoctoral nurses who are willing to undertake research training related to Alzheimer's disease and related disorders are encouraged to seek training sponsors and sites that have established research programs with this focus.

The **Health Promotion and Research Grants** emphasize basic and clinical research as it affects health promotion and illness prevention. The objective of research in this area is to decrease the vulnerability of individuals and families to illness or disability across the life span.

The **Nursing Resources for Delivery of Quality Patient Care Research Grants** support research that builds upon current knowledge about nursing resources and retention within the United States. Of special interest is research designed to examine strategies and interventions that enhance the availability and retention of RNS for the provision of quality patient care.

The **Nursing Research Specialized Centers Grants** invite applications from interested institutions, including schools of nursing or departments of nursing within appropriately staffed and grant funded clinical settings, to establish centers of excellence in nursing research devoted to the study of promising areas of patient care.

The **Nursing Research Exploratory Centers Grants** invite applications from interested institutions, including schools of nursing and departments of nursing within appropriately staffed and grant funded clinical settings, to establish exploratory, specialized centers for the study of promising areas of patient care. The exploratory grant supports feasibility studies building a base of research programs from which to compete for a specialized center in the future.

The **Nursing First Independent Research Support and Transition (FIRST Awards)** provide support for enlarging the base of scientific knowledge that underlies nursing practice, education, and services administration. FIRST awards support small studies of high quality carried out by new investigators. Via FIRST awards, new nursing investigators will develop their research capabilities and demonstrate the merit of their research ideas in new and creative ways.

For key to codes showing categories of aid, see page 17.

Specific information on the grants noted above can be obtained from Dr. Mary Leveck, Neurofunction Research; Dr. Laura James, Reproductive and Infant Health; Dr. June Lunney, Immune, Cardiopulmonary, Critical Care, Trauma, and Transplantation; Dr. Patricia Moritz, Long-Term Care and Chronic Illnesses; Dr. J. Taylor Harden, Human Development, Health and Risk Behaviors, and Women's Health, (301) 594-6869; or Sally Nichol, Grants Management Officer, (301) 594-6869; or write to: National Institute of Nursing Research, 45 Center Dr., Natcher Bldg., Bethesda, MD 20892.

The **Community-Based Prevention Intervention Research in Environmental Health Services Grants** address the development of community-based strategies aimed at prevention and intervention activities in economically disadvantaged and/or underserved populations adversely impacted by an environmental contaminant. In community-based research, active collaboration with organizations within the community that is the focus of the study are essential components of the research. These grants provide support to develop, test, and evaluate health service activities to enhance the application or transfer of existing knowledge to efforts designed to prevent or control dysfunction or disease. For specific information on this grant, contact Dr. J. Taylor Harden, Extramural Programs, (301) 594-5976, NINR; via the NIH gopher (gopher.nih.gov) and the NIH website (http://www.nih.gov); or write to the NINR at the address given above.

NATIONAL RESEARCH SERVICE AWARDS 5, 6, 7
NURSE FELLOWSHIPS
NATIONAL INSTITUTE OF NURSING RESEARCH
NATIONAL INSTITUTES OF HEALTH

The National Institute of Nursing Research now sponsors the **National Research Service Awards,** which support nurses in predoctoral and postdoctoral research training in specified areas of nursing and in certain biomedical and behavioral fields. Awards are made to (1) increase the opportunities for qualified nurses to engage in full-time study and research training; (2) prepare professional nurses to conduct independent research, collaborate in interdisciplinary research, and stimulate and guide others in nursing research;

For key to codes showing categories of aid, see page 17.

(3) promote the availability and utilization of nurses with research training in nursing or the basic sciences to function as faculty in schools of nursing; and (4) prepare nurses to conduct scientific inquiry in disciplines that have significance for nursing theory and practice.

Applicants for predoctoral study must be U.S. citizens or permanent residents and registered nurses with an active license and either a baccalaureate or master's degree in nursing. Applicants must have been admitted to a doctoral program of study and accepted by a faculty sponsor who will supervise the training and research.

Predoctoral stipends are $11,496 per year. Postdoctoral stipends range from $20,292 to $32,300, depending upon years of experience. The sponsoring institution may also receive an allowance to defray certain expenses. Appointments are made for full-time training in research. Trainees must sign a payback agreement requiring them to engage in continued nursing, biomedical, or behavioral research or teaching after completing the fellowship or to repay the amount received.

Applications are accepted at any time for inclusion in one of the three annual review cycles beginning April 5, August 5, and December 5. For more information and an application, write to: Office of Grants Inquiries, Division of Research Grants, National Institutes of Health, Bethesda, MD 20892. Telephone (301) 496-7441.

NURSES MYASTHENIA GRAVIS FELLOWSHIP   4, 5, 7

Myasthenia is a neuromuscular disease that requires skilled nursing care and observations. Fellowships are offered for research in children and adults. The fellowship allows the nurse to conduct basic research related to disease problems in patient care. The applicant must be a graduate of a baccalaureate program in nursing currently licensed as an RN, a citizen of the United States or Canada, or holding a permanent visa for training in U.S. institutions. For more information and an application, write: Executive Administrator, Myasthenia Gravis Foundation, 222 S. Riverside Plaza, Suite 1540, Chicago, IL 60606.

For key to codes showing categories of aid, see page 17.

ONCOLOGY NURSING SOCIETY/ONCOLOGY NURSING FOUNDATION   3, 5, 6, 7

The Oncology Nursing Society/Oncology Nursing Foundation are dedicated to the professional development of oncology nurses around the world. They offer numerous prestigious awards, scholarships, and research grants ranging from $1,000 to $10,000 to nurses devoted to the care of persons with cancer and to research and education in the specialty of oncology nursing. Several of the research grants include airfare to the annual Oncology Nursing Society Congress. Application deadlines vary as do the specific requirements for each award, scholarship, and research grant. For more information on each award, scholarship, and research grant offered, including specific requirements and application deadlines, contact the Oncology Nursing Society or the Oncology Nursing Foundation at 501 Holiday Drive, Pittsburgh, PA 15220-2749. Telephone (412) 921-7373.

PAN AMERICAN SANITARY BUREAU FELLOWSHIPS   7

This fellowship program intends to assist member governments in strengthening their health services; to promote cooperation among scientific groups that contribute to the advancement of health; and to improve standards of teaching and training in the health related professions. An applicant is expected to agree to work with the National Health Administration, or the institution to which he or she will be attached, for at least three years after completion of the fellowship. The government must also agree to make full use of the knowledge and experience gained by the fellow after he or she returns to her native country upon termination of the fellowship. Fellowships are open to nationals of member states of the Pan American Health Organization (PAHO) who are public health educators and workers. Fellowship applicants must be recommended by their native governments. For more information, contact: Pan American Sanitary Bureau Fellowships, Pan American Health Organization, 525 23rd Street, NW, Washington, DC 20037.

For key to codes showing categories of aid, see page 17.

REHABILITATION NURSING FOUNDATION   3, 7

The Rehabilitation Nursing Foundation (RNF) announces its annual research grant program. Funding of up to $15,000 is available and may be awarded in the form of multiple grants. A **New Investigator Award,** offered to encourage nurses who are novice researchers, will be awarded for up to $5,000. Up to two grants from the remaining funding amount will be awarded to recipients, who will be designated RNF Research Fellows.

Research proposals should address the clinical practice, educational, or administrative dimensions of rehabilitation nursing. The deadline for submission of proposals each year is April 1. Funding begins the following year for the selected proposal(s).

For a grant application or further information, please contact the RNF office at 4700 W. Lake Avenue Glenview, IL 60025. Telephone (800) 229-7530 or (847) 375-4710.

SBIR NURSING RESEARCH GRANTS   4, 5, 6, 7, 8

The **Small Business Innovation Research (SBIR) Nursing Research Grants** provide support for nurse research in, but not limited to, these areas: technology that facilitates self-care and independence of individuals with disabling conditions, clinical support systems for the improvement of patient care, research and development of new technologies for nursing care of low birth weight infants, and research and development of new technologies for nursing care of adults and children with HIV/AIDS.

Applications are open to domestic small businesses, independently owned and operated for profit, which are not dominant in the field in which research is being proposed and have no more than 500 employees. The primary employment of the principal investigator must be with the firm at the time of the award. The maximum award is for $100,000 for a six-month period for Phase I; a maximum of $750,000 is provided for a two-year period of investigation for Phase II. This SBIR Phase I Grant Solicitation and the Phase II grant application package, both text and forms, are available electronically on the NIH's "Small Business Funding Opportunities" home page at http://www.nih.gov/grants/funding/sbir.htm on the World Wide Web.

For key to codes showing categories of aid, see page 17.

Each Phase I grantee organization is entitled to submit a grant application for Phase II support either before or after expiration of the Phase I budget period. However, the Phase II application should be submitted no later than the first six receipt dates following expiration of the Phase I budget period.

A limited number of hard copies of the Phase I Grant Solicitation are produced. Subject to availability, they may be obtained from: PHS SBIR/STTR Solicitation Office, 13685 Baltimore Avenue, Laurel, MD 20707-5096. Telephone (301) 206-9696, fax (301) 206-9722, e-mail a2y@cu.nih.gov.

SUBSTANCE ABUSE AND MENTAL HEALTH 6, 7, 8
SERVICES ADMINISTRATION,
CENTER FOR MENTAL HEALTH SERVICES,
U.S. PUBLIC HEALTH SERVICE
DEPARTMENT OF HEALTH AND HUMAN SERVICES

The Center for Mental Health Services (CMHS) no longer provides direct student support. However, dependent on the availability of funds, the CMHS-sponsored program for doctoral-level mental health training in nursing is currently offered through the American Nurses Association's (ANA) Ethnic and Minority Fellowship Program. ANA should be contacted directly for up-to-date support availability information and program details.

For further general information, please write to: Carla Serlin, PhD, Director, ANA, MFP, ANA, 600 Maryland Ave SW, #100 W., Washington, DC 20024.

UNITED STATES PHARMACOPEIA FELLOWSHIP 6, 7
PROGRAM

The **United States Pharmacopeia (USP) Fellowship Program** provides twelve fellowship awards of up to $15,000. Individuals who have completed two years of full-time study in a doctoral program, are enrolled in a fellowship program, or have a post-doctoral research (non-faculty) appointment are eligible to apply.

Six fellowships will be awarded for research projects related to the standardization of drugs or other articles recognized in the

USP-NF. Six awards are available for research projects related to drug use information in the sciences and practices applicable to information handling (including information technologies) and practitioner/patient use of information on drugs and related articles recognized in the USP-DI.

A candidate's application must be endorsed by a faculty member currently serving as a member of the USP Committee of Revision or an advisory panel. Awards are made on an annual basis, and Fellows may apply for a second year of funding. Applications must be received no later than January 2 each year.

USP also offers summer intern positions to health care professions students interested in: medical and drug use information—patient education; drug product problem reporting—medication errors prevention; market research—developing promotional materials for USP products and services; and promoting USP programs through collaboration with health care organizations and through trade and public media. The summer internship is for 12 weeks. Starting and ending dates are flexible; however, all students should start on May 19 and finish on August 8. The stipend is for $6,000. A payment of $500 will be made to interns on their first day at USP to assist with relocation expenses. The remaining $5,500 will be payable on a biweekly basis over the internship. Interns are responsible for their own travel and living expenses. Applications should be received by March 1, 1997.

For further information on the USP Fellowship Program or summer intern positions, or to receive an application, contact: United States Pharmacopeia, Office of External Affairs, 12601 Twinbrook Pkwy., Rockville, MD 20852. Telephone (301) 816-8282.

W.K. KELLOGG FOUNDATION   5, 6, 7, 8
INTERNATIONAL STUDY GRANT PROGRAM
IN LATIN AMERICA AND SOUTHERN AFRICA
IN HEALTH, EDUCATION, AND AGRICULTURE

Fellowships are awarded to faculty and staff of Latin American, Caribbean, and Southern African universities, centers, institutes, foundations, councils, ministries, and departments that have active projects funded by Kellogg or where projects are being considered. The fellowship enables individuals to attend a university of choice

For key to codes showing categories of aid, see page 17.

for advanced degrees or for postgraduate studies. The individuals then return to their respective institution to teach and provide educational materials to staff, students, and clientele. Faculty and staff in nursing, primary care nursing, medicine, dentistry, allied health and health administration education, primary health care, maternal and child health, preventive medicine, and family medicine are encouraged to apply. Applicants must first be nominated by their respective place of work or study. For further information, contact: W.K. Kellogg Foundation, P.O. Box 550, Battle Creek, MI 49016-0550. Telephone (800) 819-9997.

For key to codes showing categories of aid, see page 17.

Aid from NLN's Constituent Leagues for Nursing

Many of the constituent leagues of the National League for Nursing have scholarship or loan programs to assist nursing students. This chapter describes the unique financial aid program of each constituent league that now has an awards program.

Most leagues restrict awards to residents in the geographical area that they represent and sometimes to schools in that area. Awards are sometimes limited to beginning students of nursing or to RNs, and others are available for both graduate and undergraduate study. The same numerical codes used elsewhere in this book indicate which groups of nursing students are eligible for each league's awards. The size of the awards differs among the leagues, as do the criteria for selecting recipients of awards. Since the grants the awards programs receive vary from year to year, the awards described are those for the most recent year for which information was available.

For a number of years the Schering Corporation has provided scholarship funds to the three constituent leagues that have achieved the highest percentage increase in membership. The Leagues compete with others in the same size category for the three $1,000 awards. These scholarships are awarded yearly, and are presented in alternate years at NLN's national convention.

ARIZONA LEAGUE FOR NURSING   1, 3
Public Affairs and Relations Committee
P.O. Box 85457
Tucson, AZ 85754-5457

The Arizona League for Nursing currently offers scholarships to beginning nursing students. The **Lois Pfefferbaum Memorial Scholarship** is offered in the fall to students enrolled in an RN program.
Application deadline is March 15. The **Arizona League for Nursing Scholarship** is offered in the Spring to all nursing students. Application deadline is November 15. Contact the Arizona League for
Nursing for more information on these programs.

ARKANSAS LEAGUE FOR NURSING   1, 2
11900 Cal Glenn Rd.
Little Rock, AR 72210-2820

The Arkansas League offers several scholarships for student nurses
leading to RN licensure and several scholarships for student nurses
leading to LPN licensure. Applications are mailed to schools in the
summer for selection in the fall.

CALIFORNIA LEAGUE FOR NURSING   1
851 Moreno Ave.
Palo Alto, CA 94303
Sandra MacKay, PhD, RN, Chair CLN Scholarship Committee

The California League offers three $500 scholarships to students
currently pursuing an ADN, BSN, or MSN degrees in a California
school of nursing. For more information and an application, contact
the League.

COLORADO LEAGUE FOR NURSING   1, 3, 4, 5
Sally Phillips, President
1255 S. Federal
Denver, CO 80219
(303) 270-8586

The Colorado League awards several scholarships each to state residents enrolled in an NLN-accredited school of nursing in Colorado

For key to codes showing categories of aid, see page 17.

who show proof of good academic standing and unmet financial need. Students may apply to eligible schools for applications, which detail times for submission; recipients are determined by the Colorado League's Scholarship Committee. Winners are announced at CLN's annual meeting, and awards are paid directly to the school where the recipient is enrolled.

CONNECTICUT LEAGUE FOR NURSING   1, 3, 4
P.O. Box 365
Wallingford, CT 06492-0365

Scholarships are awarded to Connecticut residents enrolled in an NLN-accredited school of nursing which is also a CLN agency member. All applicants must satisfy the following criteria per their course of study: baccalaureate applicants must have completed the 3rd year of a 4-year program; diploma applicants must have completed the 1st year of a 2-year program; associate degree applicants must have completed the first year of a 2-year program; RN students in an upper-division BSN program must be entering the senior year of the nursing program; and graduate students must have completed 20 credits in an accredited nursing program. Deadline for applications is October 15.

DISTRICT OF COLUMBIA LEAGUE FOR   3, 4, 5
NURSING
P.O. Box 57152
Washington, DC 20037-7152
(202) 728-2956

The District of Columbia League offers one to four scholarships annually for nurses who are licensed to practice in the District of Columbia. The award is for $500 and is granted to RNs who are pursuing a BSN, MSN, or doctoral degree at an NLN-accredited school of nursing in the District of Columbia. Contact the District of Columbia League for more information about this award.

FLORIDA LEAGUE FOR NURSING   3, 5, 7
P.O. Box 533377
Orlando, FL 32853-3377

The Florida League for Nursing offers scholarships for RN to BSN and RN to MSN nursing and graduate students who are residents of Florida. Research grants are awarded for Florida League for Nursing members only. Contact the Florida League for Nursing for more information on these programs.

GEORGIA LEAGUE FOR NURSING   1, 3, 5, 6
1362 W. Peachtree St.
Atlanta, GA 30309
(404) 874-4068

The Georgia League currently offers three scholarships to advance nursing education. The **Spilman-Bischoff Nursing Scholarship** is a $1,000 award for a graduate nurse enrolled in a master's or doctoral program at an NLN-accredited institution and preparing to practice in Georgia. Preference will be given to applicants who are members of the Georgia League for Nursing and demonstrate need and evidence of leadership.

The **Lucy Willard Scholarship** is a $500 award for undergraduate students currently enrolled in the nursing course sequence of an NLN-accredited nursing program in Georgia. Priority is given to current members of the League or to members of the Georgia Association of Nursing Students.

The **Sarah Helen Killgore Scholarship** is a $500 award for undergraduate study in an NLN-accredited nursing program in Georgia. Applicants must be currently enrolled in the nursing course sequence and must maintain a GPA of 3.0. Priority is given to current members of the League or to members of the Georgia Association of Nursing Students.

Applications may be obtained from the Financial Aid Office of the school where the student is enrolled or from the Georgia League of Nursing office. Winners of awards are determined by the Scholarship Committee of the Georgia League for Nursing. Scholarships are renewable for subsequent years of study as applicable.

ILLINOIS LEAGUE FOR NURSING 1, 5
P.O. Box 597378
Chicago, IL 60659

The Illinois League for Nursing offers scholarship awards for beginning RN studies and special research grants. For more information on scholarships offered contact the Illinois League for Nursing.

INDIANA LEAGUE FOR NURSING 1, 2, 3, 5
2915 N. High School Rd.
Indianapolis, IN 46203

The Indiana League offers graduate and undergraduate scholarships for nursing students. Applicants must be residents of Indiana and attend an NLN-accredited school of nursing. For more information, contact the Indiana League directly.

IOWA LEAGUE FOR NURSING 1, 3, 5
P.O. Box 1202 Welch Post Office
Ames, IA 50014

Any associate degree, diploma, baccalaureate, or master's nursing student who attends an Iowa school and has at least a C average and financial need may apply for the Iowa League Scholarship. Awards depend on the availability of funds. Applicants need not be Iowa residents. Criteria for the scholarship include (1) academic standing, (2) financial need, and (3) personal qualifications. The application must be signed by the director of the school of nursing where the applicant attends. The deadline for application is June 1, and students are notified in August.

KENTUCKY LEAGUE FOR NURSING 1, 2, 3, 4, 5
P.O. Box 574
Murray, KY 42071

The Kentucky League awards several scholarships. The criteria for eligibility are high grade point average, good character, and favorable references. Requests for applications may be addressed to the President, Kentucky League for Nursing at the above address; applicants will be notified of a deadline date. The award is presented at the annual meeting of the Kentucky League.

For key to codes showing categories of aid, see page 17.

LOUISIANA LEAGUE FOR NURSING   5
Joan Nasser
Louisiana League for Nursing
1900 Gravier Street, Second Floor #2A9
New Orleans, LA 70112
FAX (504) 568-8295
Phone (504) 899-3193

The Louisiana League offers one scholarship per year for a nursing student pursuing graduate (master's or doctoral) studies. Applicants must be Louisiana residents and members of the League. For more information, contact the Louisiana League.

MASSACHUSETTS/RHODE ISLAND LEAGUE   1, 2, 3
FOR NURSING
1 Thompson Square
Charlestown, MA 02129

This constituent league awards scholarships for undergraduate study (RN completion, entering or in final year of generic program, and practical nursing study after fourth month). For an undergraduate award, applicants must be residents of Massachusetts or Rhode Island for a minimum of four (4) years and show financial need, satisfactory scholarship, and an ability to contribute to nursing. Awards may be paid either to the student or directly to schools. For PN students, completed applications must be received by January 31 and recipient(s) only are notified by March 15. For RN students, completed applications must be received by July 15 and recipient(s) only are notified by August 15.

Address requests for applications to MARILN Scholarship Committee at the above address (include a 55 cent stamped business-sized self-addressed envelope).

MICHIGAN LEAGUE FOR NURSING   1, 2, 3
33150 Schoolcraft Road, Suite 201
Livonia, MI 48150-1646
(313) 427-1900

The Michigan League for Nursing offers scholarship awards to selected applicants each year. All applicants must be currently enrolled in an undergraduate nursing program, have successfully completed at least one clinical nursing course with a 2.0 or higher and present endorsement by one faculty member. Awards winners will be selected based on completion of an application and an essay to be judged by the MLN Council on Nursing Education. The amount of awards depends on the number of winners and available funds. The application deadline is February 15th each year. Awards will be presented in early spring of each year during the MLN Annual Conference and Membership Meeting. For an application write directly to the Michigan League for Nursing.

MINNESOTA LEAGUE FOR NURSING   3, 4, 5
P.O. Box 24713
Edina, MN 55424
(612) 829-5891

The Minnesota League for Nursing, in cooperation with the American Cancer Society, offers four $1,500 awards to be given in the fall of 1996. Two awards each are to be offered to undergraduate and graduate students living in or attending school in the State of Minnesota. The **Undergraduate** award will be given to either a junior or senior nursing student in a BA/BS nursing program. The applicant may be either a full-time or part-time student in a generic or RN degree completion program. The **Graduate** award will be given to an individual in a master's or doctorate in nursing program. For more information on these awards, contact the Minnesota League for Nursing.

MISSOURI LEAGUE FOR NURSING   1, 2, 3, 4, 5
P.O. Box 104476
Jefferson City, MO 65110-4476

The Missouri League for Nursing has three scholarships for Missouri residents attending NLN-accredited schools of nursing. The **MLN Margo Ballard Memorial Scholarship** is available to LPN students, RN students above the freshman level in associate and diploma programs and above the sophomore level in baccalaureate programs, and MSN students who have completed at least 15 hours of courses required for the advanced degree and are licensed in Missouri.

The **Vivian Meinecke Scholarship** is available to practical and professional nursing students above the freshman level in associate and diploma programs and above the sophomore level in baccalaureate nursing programs.

The **Missouri League for Nursing Scholarships** are available to LPN students, RN students above the freshman level in associate degree/diploma programs and above the sophomore level in baccalaureate nursing programs, and MSN students who have completed at least 15 hours of courses required for the advanced degree and are licensed in Missouri. This award may be distributed to more than one candidate.

Applications must be submitted by nursing schools in Missouri, each of which may send in only one application per scholarship, no later than November 1. The Missouri League for Nursing Scholarship Committee chooses the winners based on personal qualifications, including extracurricular activities in nursing, academic qualification, and financial need. Winners are notified by December 1. These scholarships are not renewable, but winners may reapply. The amount of each award varies. A student who receives an award and does not complete the semester for which a grant is made must return the entire amount.

NEBRASKA LEAGUE FOR NURSING   1, 3
Jeanette Ekberg
Scholarship Committee Chair
4707 Manchester
Omaha, NE 68152

The Nebraska League for Nursing offers scholarships for nursing students pursuing baccalaureate, RN, and LPN studies. For more information, contact the Nebraska League for Nursing.

NEW JERSEY LEAGUE FOR NURSING   1, 3
332 North Avenue
Garwood, NJ 07027
(908) 789-3398

The New Jersey League awards several scholarships to senior students attending an NLN-accredited school of nursing within New Jersey. State residency is required. Awards are granted on the basis of merit, financial need, and scholastic ability.

Applications must be made in writing and may be obtained from the New Jersey League office, marked to the attention of the Scholarship Committee. Completed applications are due back April 30th with awards issued in July for the following semester. With the application include an official school transcript, references, and a personal statement from the applicant.

NEW MEXICO LEAGUE FOR NURSING   1, 2, 3
Scholarship Committee
P.O. Box 40186
Albuquerque, NM 87192

The New Mexico League for Nursing offers scholarships annually for New Mexico residents currently enrolled in any NLN-accredited nursing program in New Mexico at the undergraduate or master's level. The scholarships vary in amount, and applicants must have been enrolled in their present program for at least one successful trimester. Applications are due each Spring.

WESTERN NEW YORK LEAGUE FOR NURSING   3, 5
Sharon L. Davt
Board of Directors
4873 Sunway Lane
Hamburg, NY 14075

In memory of Lucretia H. Richter, the Western New York League is scheduled to award three $1,000 scholarships in 1996–1997. The criteria for awards are enrollment in an NLN-accredited RN program in the region, commitment to professional nursing, financial need, and satisfactory academic and clinical standing. Specific awards and applications may be obtained from NLN-accredited schools in the region from October 15 to December 1. For the January 1997 awards, the application deadline is December 1, 1996. Faculty recommendation is required. Please contact the Western New York League for the current status and scholarship award offerings.

For key to codes showing categories of aid, see page 17.

NORTH CAROLINA LEAGUE FOR NURSING   3, 5
c/o Dr. Ruby G. Barnes, Chairman
Academic Scholarship Committee
1622 Village Glen Drive
Raleigh, NC 27612-4340

The North Carolina League for Nursing offers scholarship awards for baccalaureate completion and graduate study for RNs. For more information on scholarships offered contact the North Carolina League for Nursing.

OHIO LEAGUE FOR NURSING   1, 2
Cleveland Area
2800 Euclid Avenue, Suite 235
Cleveland, OH 44115

This constituent league made numerous awards in the last academic year, for a total of almost $20,000 in the form of grants, loans, and combination grant/loans. The size of individual awards ranged between $400 and $1,000, depending on the level of study and the cost of the program, as well as need. Funds for the financial aid program are derived from foundation grants, a revolving loan fund, and an endowment.

Applicants must be residents of Cuyahoga, Geauga, Lake, Portage, Medina, Summit, or Lorain counties in Ohio, and must have completed one clinical nursing course and have a 3.0 average. LPN applicants should provide a post-secondary transcript if possible. All awards are for full-time study. Recipients of awards must agree to practice nursing in a health care facility in the seven-county area for at least one year after completion of the program.

Applications may be obtained from the Ohio League and are due back by April 30th, along with two references plus a 1040 form. The Financial Aid Committee determines the recipients on the basis of financial need and scholarship. Students may reapply for awards each year.

Repayment of loans begins 90 days after completion of the nursing program at a fixed rate of interest. If the recipient of a grant does not complete the program of study, the monies must be repaid under the same terms as loan monies.

Recipients of awards are notified by mid-July of the amount and type of award and are advised to present the letter to the school's financial aid officer who will bill the Ohio League. Awards are paid directly to the school and applied to tuition, unless a student has special needs, in which case some of the award can be applied to school-related expenses, such as books, uniforms, or fees.

OKLAHOMA LEAGUE FOR NURSING   1, 2, 3, 4
P.O. Box 26068
Oklahoma City, OK 73126

The Oklahoma League for Nursing awards several scholarships annually in March for students seeking education in Oklahoma. Contact the League for more information concerning this scholarship.

OREGON LEAGUE FOR NURSING   1, 3, 4, 5
16740 N.W. Yorktown Dr.
Beaverton, OR 97006

The Oregon League offers scholarships for nursing students pursuing associate, baccalaureate, master's, or doctoral degrees. The **Ella McKinney Fund** provides at least two scholarships of up to $500 for nursing students. The **OCNEN Fund** provides scholarships of up to $700 for nurses who require financial assistance while attending continuing education programs. For more information and applications, contact the Oregon League.

PENNSYLVANIA LEAGUE FOR NURSING   1, 2, 3, 5
PLN Awards and Scholarship Committee
Pennsylvania League for Nursing, Inc.
660 Lonely Cottage Drive
Upper Black Eddy, PA 18972-9313

Each year the Pennsylvania League for Nursing (PLN) offers one $500 scholarship (RN) and one $250 scholarship (LPN). Applicants for either scholarship must be Pennsylvania residents, attend an accredited program, and currently be enrolled on a part-time or full-time basis. Applicants for the $500 scholarship must be in the final year of study if enrolled in a diploma, associate degree, BSN,

BSN-RN, or masters program. Doctoral candidates must have completed all course work and be prepared to submit an annual progress report if graduation does not occur in one year. All applicants must submit a letter of endorsement from the Director of their educational program along with the application form.

SOUTH CAROLINA LEAGUE FOR NURSING   1, 3, 5
1159 Shilling Place
Mt. Pleasant, SC 29464

The South Carolina League for Nursing offers scholarships for beginning RN study and for baccalaureate completion for RNs. Contact the League for more information on these scholarships. South Carolina residents only may apply.

TEXAS LEAGUE FOR NURSING   7
Patty Roberts
P.O. Box 80110
Austin, TX 78708-0110

The Texas League for Nursing offers three awards every two years at its biennial convention. The **Teaching Excellence Award** is given to recognize quality teaching in schools of nursing, in health care facilities, and in the community. The **Nursing Research Award** is presented to an individual whose research makes significant contributions to nursing practice and health care in Texas. The recipient of this award must be able to present his or her research at the TLN Biennial Convention. The **Nursing Excellence in Community Health Award** honors nurses who have made contributions to nursing in community-based settings through commitment to patient care, education and community service. All award honorees receive a cash award and commemorative plaque.

VIRGINIA LEAGUE FOR NURSING/VIRGINIA   1
NURSING STUDENTS' ASSOCIATION
Brenda Nichols, Scholarship Chair
676 Green Valley Drive
Virginia Beach, VA 23962

The Virginia League for Nursing offers six to ten awards of $400 each to nursing students who are residents of Virginia. Applicants

For key to codes showing categories of aid, see page 17.

also must be attending a school of nursing in Virginia and be a member of NSNA. Awards are made directly to the student for educationally related expenses. These awards are considered outright grants providing the recipient completes the nursing program. The VNSA offers additional scholarships using the same applications and criteria as VLN.

WASHINGTON LEAGUE FOR NURSING   1, 3, 5
Dr. Sandra Eyres
Professor
University of Washington
School of Nursing
Seattle, Washington 98195

In 1993, the Washington League for Nursing initiated the awarding of two annual scholarships of $500 each to a nursing student (graduate or undergraduate) who is a resident of Washington. Criteria for selection are: (1) full-time enrollment in an NLN-accredited nursing program, (2) excellent academic standing, and (3) evidence of leadership qualities.

Application forms may be requested at the above address. All completed forms must be accompanied by a copy of the school transcript and two recommendations that address the selection criteria. An appointed committee reviews all applications, and scholarships are presented to award winners at an annual meeting of the Washington League.

WEST VIRGINIA LEAGUE FOR NURSING   1, 3
169 Tartan Drive
Fallansbee, WV 26037

The West Virginia League for Nursing awards grants to second, third, or fourth year students attending a West Virginia school of nursing when funds are available. Contact the League for further information.

WISCONSIN LEAGUE FOR NURSING   1, 5
2121 East Newport Ave.
Milwaukee, WI 53211

The WLN has a long history of awarding scholarships. Currently this constituent league annually awards eight to ten scholarships of $500 each with funds obtained from foundations and corporate grants and from fund raising drives. Wisconsin students who study in a Wisconsin NLN accredited basic RN or graduate program and who have completed at least one half of program requirements, are eligible for these awards. Application forms are sent to deans of schools in Wisconsin for their distribution. The WLN Scholarship Committee members determine the winners after considering need and academics. Winners are notified and asked to attend the Scholarship Luncheon usually in April. Deadlines for applications vary from year to year.

The WLN also offers one $500 scholarship to a high school senior resident of Wisconsin and already accepted by a NLN Wisconsin accredited School of Nursing. Seniors are asked to contact the WLN direct for an application.

WYOMING LEAGUE FOR NURSING   1, 2, 3, 4, 5
125 College Drive
Casper, WY 82601
(307)268-2235

Scholarships are awarded to students pursuing the RN or LPN degree. Applicants must be currently enrolled in an NLN-accredited nursing education program in the state of Wyoming. Along with the completed application, a letter of recommendation from a current faculty member is required. Contact the League for more information and application forms.

Resources

Much of the financial aid described in this book, aside from the federal aid for undergraduates, is specific for nursing education and research. Many other sources exist, and the references listed below will guide you in finding them. The inexpensive pamphlets *Don't Miss Out* and *Need a Lift?* will open your eyes to the myriad organizations and agencies that give money for education. Religious groups, unions, fraternal, social and nationality organizations, and employers often have scholarships or loans for members and their families. Many corporations have special-purpose scholarships. Be certain to write your state's education agency and call your local chamber of commerce for information about grants and scholarships.

The more expensive publications listed here are reference books and should be found in a public or school library. The list could be much longer. If you are serious in your ambition to become a nurse or to advance your nursing career educationally or by research, and if you are willing to put time and effort into exploring available sources, you are certain to find ways to help finance your goal!

Annual Register of Grant Support: A Directory of Funding Sources.
R.R. Bowker, a division of Reed Elsevier, 121 Chanlon Rd., New Providence, NJ 07974. Telephone (908) 464-6800. 1997 edition, $199.95. Over 3,200 listings of grants, fellowships, and awards in various fields.

The A's and B's of Academic Scholarships. Octameron Associates, P.O. Box 2748, Alexandria, VA 22301. Updated annually, $9 (postpaid). Listings of academic scholarships from individual colleges and universities and some other sources. For undergraduate studies only.

111

The Big Book of Minority Opportunities. Edited by Willis L. Johnson. Garrett Park Press, Garrett Park, MD 20896. 1995 edition, $39 plus $3 for shipping and handling. Lists over 2,900 general programs of interest to minority group members, including national, regional, and area scholarship programs, employment services, special academic programs, and job banks, plus federal programs and aid offered by individual colleges and universities.

Chronicle Financial Aid Guide. Chronicle Guidance Publications, Inc., 66 Aurora Street, P.O. Box 1190, Moravia, NY 13118-1190. $22.47 plus $2.50 shipping and handling. Order No. 502A. Revised annually. Information on more than 1,600 financial aid programs for high school seniors, college undergraduates, and adult learners from private corporations, labor unions, federal government, and state education agencies. A Subject Index gives easy access to programs by majors for which students may be eligible. 1997–1998 edition available fall 1997.

The College Blue Book: Scholarships, Fellowships, Grants, and Loans. Macmillan Library Reference, 1633 Broadway, 5th Floor, New York, NY 10019-6785. $48. This volume of The College Blue Book is arranged by area of interest and includes 80 separate nursing scholarships.

The College Cost Book. College Board Publications, Box 886, New York, NY 10101. Annual. 1996–1997 edition, $16.95. A step-by-step guide for determining college costs (including worksheets) and applying for financial aid. Outlines major aid programs and lists current costs at more than 3,100 institutions.

College Financial Aid for Dummies, by Dr. Herm Davis and Joyce Lain Kennedy. IDG Books Worldwide, 919 E. Hillsdale Boulevard, Suite 400, Foster City, CA 94404. Internet: www.dummies.com, $16.95. A how-to book for 1998–1999 school year with scholarships for both traditional and nontraditional (adults, part-timers, distance ed, international students and U.S. students abroad) stude.

The College Financial Aid Emergency Kit. By Joyce Lain Kennedy and Dr. Herm Davis. Sun Features, Inc., Box 368, Cardiff, CA

92007. 1997–1998 edition, $6.40 plus 55 postage ($6.95 total). Comprehensive pocket guide to applying for financial aid.

Directory of Biomedical and Health Care Grants is an important resource in tracking large grant-making institutional awards to individuals, universities, colleges, nonprofit organizations, hospitals, and other health-care-related institutions. This resource is commonly found in public, college, and university libraries.

Directory of Financial Aid for Minorities (1995–1997). $47.50 plus $4.50 shipping and handling. A thorough source for available financial aid for minorities. More than 2,000 funding opportunities are described. Reference Service Press, 1100 Industrial Road, Suite 9, San Carlos, CA 94070.

Directory of Financial Aids for Women, 1997–1999 edition. By Gail A. Schlachter, Reference Service Press, 5000 Windplay Drive, Suite 4, El Dorado Hills, CA 95762. $45, plus $4.50 shipping. Identifies more than 1,800 scholarships, fellowships, grants, loans, awards, and internships set aside for women and women's organizations.

Don't Miss Out: The Ambitious Student's Guide to Financial Aid. By Robert Leider and Anna Leider. Octameron Associates, Inc., P.O. Box 2748, Alexandria, VA 22301. Updated annually, $9 (postpaid). Explains how to calculate college costs and family contribution, and offers advice on different routes to explore for assistance depending on your abilities and interests. Section on aid for health careers, minorities, and women.

Encyclopedia of Associations: International Organizations. Gale Research, Inc., 835 Penobscot Building, Detroit, MI 48226. 1997 edition is available now and the 1998 edition will be available July 11, 1997. Reference guide to more than 19,400 multinational, binational, and national organizations in more than 200 countries. $550. On-line data offered. Telephone (800) 877-GALE.

Encyclopedia of Associations: National Organizations of the U.S. Gale Research, 835 Penobscot Building, Detroit, MI 48226. 32nd edition. Reference source for comprehensive listings and descriptions of national organizations, nonprofit groups, fraternal organizations, and other groups in three volumes: Volume 1, National Organizations of the U.S., $460; Volume 2, Geographic and Executive Indexes, $355; Volume 3, Supplement, $390. On-line data offered. Telephone (800) 877-GALE.

Encyclopedia of Associations: Regional, State and Local Organizations. Gale Research, Inc., 835 Penobscot Building, Detroit, MI 48226. 1997 edition. Reference guide to nonprofit membership organizations with interstate, state, intrastate, city or local scope and interest. Five volumes at $30 per volume; $125 per entire set. On-line data offered. Telephone (800) 877-GALE.

Financial Advice for Minority Students Seeking an Education in the Health Professions. An informative brochure for minority students. Free. Health Professions Career Opportunity Program, 1600 Ninth Street, Room 441, Sacramento, CA 95814.

Financial Aid for Minorities in Health Fields. Garrett Park Press, P.O. Box 190F, Garrett Park, MD 20896. Annual, $5.90 per booklet plus $1.50 shipping and handling. Summary of employment outlook and the number of minority members in each field, directory of several hundred financial aid programs, list of associations or organizations in each field, and resources for supplementary information.

Foundation Grants to Individuals, New 10th edition. Foundation Center, 79 Fifth Avenue, New York, NY 10003. $65 plus $4.50 for shipping. An important source for independent and corporate foundations that award grants to individuals. It is also an important source for undergraduate and graduate scholarships, fellowships, research grants, residencies, internships, and grants offered by U.S. foundations; includes company-sponsored aid.

Health Professions Education Directory: 1997–1998. American Medical Association, 515 N State St., Chicago, IL 60610. 1996–1997 edition, $54.95 plus $11.95 shipping and handling. Provides information on nearly 5,000 health education programs sponsored by more than 2,200 institutions. Covers 41 health careers, including dental-related, dietetic, and audiology/speech language pathology occupations, accredited by 12 national agencies. Also includes data on enrollment, graduation, and attrition for most occupations. To place orders, call (800) 621-8335 or fax (312) 464-5830. For more information, contact Fred Donini-Lenhoff at (312) 464-4635.

Loans and Grants From Uncle Sam: Am I Eligible and for How Much? Octameron Associates, P.O. Box 2748, Alexandria, VA 22301. Updated annually, $6 (postpaid). Explains whether you're eligible for federal grants and loans and how to decide which of the many forms of loans from the federal government are appropriate for you.

National Guide to Funding in Health is an important resource in tracking large grant-making institutional awards to individuals, universities, colleges, nonprofit organizations, and other health-care-related institutions. This resource is commonly found in public, college, and university libraries.

Need a Lift? Emblem Sales, P.O. Box 1050, Indianapolis, IN 46206. Annual. 1997 edition, $3 (prepaid). Lists sources of aid for all students, including federal and state programs, private sources, and student employment and cooperative education programs, as well as aid offered by The American Legion and sources of assistance for veterans and their dependents.

Scholarship Directory 1997–1998 Minority Guide to Scholarships and Financial Aid. A valuable directory to scholarships and financial aid for minorities. $7 plus $.98 shipping. Tinsley Communications, Inc., 100 Bridge Street, Suite A-3, Hampton, VA 23669.

Scholarships, Fellowships and Loans. Gale Research, 835 Penobscot Building, 645 Griswold, Detroit, MI 48226. 1997 edition. $155. Contains listings of information about financial aid for students at all levels of study in the United States and Canada, cross-referenced by vocational goals, field of study, legal residence, place of study, special recipient, and organization and award indexes. Includes many national and state sources for nursing. Telephone (800) 877-GALE.

A Selected List of Fellowship Opportunities and Aids to Advanced Education for United States Citizens and Foreign Nationals. National Science Foundation, Publications Office, 1800 G Street, NW, Room 232, Washington, DC 20550. Free. Lists over 100 fellowships for advanced study in various fields.

Sources of Financial Aid Available to American Indian Students. $4. A helpful guide to current financial aid awards available to American Indian students. Indian Resource Development, New Mexico State University, Box 30001, Department 3 IRD, Las Cruces, NM 88003.

NLN CAREER PUBLICATIONS

Annual Guide to Graduate Nursing Education Program 1996. From the Center for Research in Nursing Education and Community Health. Pub No. 19-6924, $27.95. The definitive listing of master's and doctoral level nursing programs in the United States and its territories.

Career Planning: A Nurse's Guide to Career Advancement. By Patricia Winstead-Frey, PhD, RN. Pub. No. 41-2295, $16.50. A revealing text for career development courses, as an aid in recruitment, and as a self-help manual for nurses interested in pursuing careers outside of the traditional hospital setting.

Entrepreneuring: A Nurse's Guide to Starting a Business, 2nd Edition. By Gerry Vogel, MSN, RN, and Nancy Doleysh, MSN, RN. Pub. No. 14-2635, $24.95. A practical guide to career enhancement through entrepreneuring in health care, including: ventures in clinical practices, consulting, home care, product support, and much more.

Managing Your Career in Nursing, 2nd Edition. By Frances C. Henderson, EdD, RN, and Barbara O. McGettigan, MS, RN. Pub. No. 14-2640, $25.95. A "mentor-in-print" for any nurse who wants to take a practical, self-directed approach to lifelong career management. Community nursing, self-employment, informatics, nursing research, education and administration, and new nursing roles are covered. Perfect for new graduates, current or prospective nursing students, guidance counselors, and development professionals.

The NLN Guide to Undergraduate RN Education. From the Center for Research in Nursing Education and Community Health. Pub. No. 41-6797, $19.95. A handbook on pursuing a nursing career combined with a state-by-state directory of NLN-accredited schools of nursing is available to high school and college students, guidance counselors, and anyone considering a career in nursing.

Nursing: The Career of a Lifetime. By Shirley H. Fondiller, EdD, RN, FAAN, and B. J. Nerone, APR. Pub. No. 14-2695, $19.95. The most current, all-inclusive guide to nursing as a life-long career. Professional options are thoroughly explored for all levels of nursing students and licensed practitioners in this state-of-the-art resource.

On Doctoral Education in Nursing: The Voice of the Student By Dona Rinaldi Carpenter, EdD, RN, CS, and Sharon Hudacek, EdD, RN, CS. Pub. No. 14-6703, $27.95. Doctoral candidates in nursing face a range of confusing choices. Choosing the best program that meets your particular criteria can be a harrowing experience. Now, you can learn from the mistakes and successes of the diverse range of doctoral students and educators in PhD, EdD, and DNS programs. In their own words, they reveal the pitfalls and pratfalls they have faced and overcome, looking at how economic difficulties, family responsibilities, and long hours have affected their education. Essential for anyone considering pursuing a doctoral degree in nursing.

NLN VIDEOS

Career Encounters: Advanced Practice Nursing
A comprehensive video overview of the career options available to RNs. The perfect tool for nurse educators, nursing directors, guidance counselors, recruiters and students.

From this series of intimate and moving interviews, viewers will discover the challenges and rewards of the field, and learn what qualities and skills make a good candidate for an APN program. Purchase: ½″ VHS (Pub. No. 42-2659): $175. 10-Day Rental $75 (42-2659R). 30 minutes.

Career Encounters: Nursing

Developed by the NLN in collaboration with David Gray, Inc. and co-sponsored by the Veteran's Administration, this video presents an intimate look at nursing through the eyes of successful nursing professionals. Meet the founder of a profitable nursing business, a critical care nurse in a city hospital, a home health nurse caring for patients with AIDS, and many others.

The program offers a special career guidance section which helps viewers match their own character and work style to the variety of jobs available within nursing, including printed supplementary material detailing additional nursing career information and resources. 27 minutes.
Purchase: ½″ VHS (Pub. No. 42-2380): $125

Center for Career Advancement

This service of the National League for Nursing can help you find the nursing program you are looking for with a customized computer search that matches your individual needs to a specific program, including LPN, undergraduate and graduate level. For questions or to order a search, call the Center for Career Advancement at (800) 669-1656, ext. 472.

How to Start a Nursing Center

Nursing centers offer Americans a radically different model of health care, combining high quality and accessibility with low cost. *How to Start a Nursing Center* is the only video that tells you how to get started in a variety of settings—from academic to freestanding.

The video contains all the information you need to open a center, including: planning services, funding, making faculty practice arrangements, and ensuring profitability. Success stories from nursing centers at Emory University and Arizona State University, as well as from a freestanding midwifery center are presented. The

video also reports pertinent new findings from NLN's national survey of nursing centers and includes an extensive list of funding sources. 34 minutes.
Purchase: ½" VHS (Pub. No. 42-2502): $87.50

The Power of Nursing

The Power of Nursing discusses the nature of power and offers viewers a rare glimpse into the private and professional lives of three women who began their careers as staff nurses and became outstanding national leaders. Their outlooks, accomplishments, and guiding principles are a unique catalyst for personal and professional change.

In *The Power of Nursing*, Sheila Burke, Chief of Staff, Office of the Republican Leader; Rae Grad, Executive Director, National Commission to Prevent Infant Mortality; and Maria Mitchell, Former President and Chief Operating Officer, CHAP, identify the components of power and explain how to use it effectively. The video is a springboard for individual introspection and follow-up discussion. Moreover, it is a dynamic educational resource and motivational tool. 25 minutes.
Purchase: ½" VHS (Pub. No. 42-2452): $100

Any of these NLN videos or publications may be ordered from: Customer Service, National League for Nursing, 350 Hudson Street, New York, NY 10014. All orders must be prepaid. Institutional orders can be billed when accompanied by an authorized purchase order. Please add $3.95 for shipping and handling charges for orders up to $24.99, and $5.55 for orders over $25. For orders over $100, add $8.15 for shipping and handling charges.

Appendix

DIRECTORY OF BOARDS OF NURSING

Judi Crume, Exec. Off.
Board of Nursing
P.O. Box 303900
Montgomery, AL 36130-3900
Tel.: (205) 242-4060

Dorothy Fulton, Exec. Sec.
Alaska Board of Nursing
3601 C St., Suite 722
Anchorage, AK 99503
Tel.: (907) 561-2878

Marie Mao, Exec. Sec.
Health Services Regulatory Board
LBJ Tropical Medical Center
Pago Pago, American Samoa
  96799
Tel.: (684) 633-1222

Joey Ridemour, Exec. Dir.
Arizona State Board of Nursing
1651 E. Morton, Suite 150
Phoenix, AZ 85020
Tel.: (602) 255-5092

Faith Fields, Exec. Dir.
Arkansas State Board of Nursing
1123 South University, Suite 800
Little Rock, AR 72204
Tel.: (501) 686-2700

Ruth Terry, Exec. Off.
Board of Registered Nursing
P.O. Box 944210
Sacramento, CA 94244-2100
Tel.: (213) 897-3590

Karen Brumley, Prog. Admin.
Colorado State Board of Nursing
1560 Broadway, Suite 670
Denver, CO 82002-2410
Tel.: (303) 894-2430

Dr. Marie Hilliard, Exec. Off.
Department of Public Health
410 Capitol Ave., Box 340308
Hartford, CT 06134-0308
Tel.: (860) 509-7624

Iva Boardman, Exec. Dir.
Delaware Board of Nursing
Cannon Bldg., P.O. Box 1401
Dover, DE 19901
Tel.: (302) 739-4522

Barbara Hagans, Contact
  Representative
District of Columbia Board of
  Nursing
614 H St. N.W.
Washington, DC 20013
Tel.: (202) 727-7856

121

Marilyn Bloss, Exec. Dir.
Florida State Board of Nursing
4080 Woodcock Dr.
Jacksonville, FL 32201
Tel.: (904) 798-4215

Shirley Camp, Exec. Dir.
Georgia Board of Nursing
166 Pryor St., S.W.
Atlanta, GA 30334
Tel.: (404) 656-5167

Teofila P. Cruz, Exec. Dir.
Guam Board of Nurse Examiners
P.O. Box 2816
Agana, Guam 96910
Tel.: (671) 734-7295

Kathleen Yokouchi, Exec. Off.
Hawaii Board of Nursing
Box 3469
Honolulu, HI 99503
Tel.: (808) 586-2695

Sandra Evans, Asst. Exec. Dir.
Idaho State Board of Nursing
P.O. Box 83720
Boise, ID 83720-0061
Tel.: (208) 334-3110

Elizabeth Cleinmark, Acting
  Coord.
Department of Professional
  Regulations
320 W. Washington St.
Springfield, IL 62786
Tel.: (217) 785-9465

Gina Voorhies, Dir.
Indiana State Board of Nursing
402 W. Washington St.
Indianapolis, IN 46204
Tel.: (317) 233-4405

Lorinda Inman, Exec. Dir.
Iowa Board of Nursing
1223 E. Court Ave.
Des Moines, IA 50319
Tel.: (515) 281-4828

Pat Johnson, Exec. Admin.
Kansas State Board of Nursing
900 S.W. Jackson St., Suite 551S
Topeka, KS 66612-1256
Tel.: (913) 296-3782

Sharon M. Weisenbeck, Exec. Dir.
Kentucky Board of Nursing
312 Whittington Pky., Suite 300
Louisville, KY 40222-5172
Tel.: (502) 329-7000

Barbara Morvant, Exec. Dir.
Louisiana State Board of Nursing
3510 N. Causeway Blvd.,
  Suite 501
Metairie, LA 70002-3531
Tel.: (504) 838-5332

Jean C. Carson, Exec. Dir.
Maine State Board of Nursing
35 Anthony Ave.
State House Station 158
Augusta, ME 04333-0158
Tel.: (207) 287-1133

Donna Dorsey, Exec. Dir.
Maryland Board of Nursing
4140 Patterson Ave.
Baltimore, MD 21215-2254
Tel.: (301) 764-5124

Theresa M. Bonanno, Exec. Sec.
Board of Registration in Nursing
100 Cambridge St., Rm. 150
Boston, MA 02202
Tel.: (617) 727-3060

Mary Vandenbosch, Nurse
Consultant
Michigan Board of Nursing
P.O. Box 30018
611 West Ottawa
Lansing, MI 48909
Tel.: (517) 373-4674

Joyce M. Schowalter, Exec. Dir.
Minnesota Board of Nursing
2700 University Ave., W. 108
St. Paul, MN 55114
Tel.: (612) 643-2565

Ann Homer Cook, Assoc.
Commissioner
Institution of Higher Learning
3825 Ridgewood Rd.
Jackson, MS 39211
Tel.: (601) 982-6690

Florence Stillman, Exec. Dir.
Missouri State Board of Nursing
3605 Missouri Blvd.
Jefferson City, MO 65102
Tel.: (573) 751-0080

Dianne Wickham, Exec. Dir.
Montana State Board of Nursing
Arcade Bldg.—111 Jackson
Helena, MT 59620-0513
Tel.: (406) 444-2071

Dr. Charlene Kelly, Assoc. Dir.
Bureau of Examining Bd.
P.O. Box 95007
Lincoln, NE 68509
Tel.: (402) 471-4917

Kathy Apple, Exec. Dir.
Nevada State Board of Nursing
4335 S. Industrial Rd. #430
Las Vegas, NV 89103
Tel.: (702) 739-1575

Doris G. Nuttelman, Exec. Dir.
State Board of Nursing
Div. of Public Health
6 Hazen Dr.
Concord, NH 03301
Tel.: (603) 271-2323

Harriet Johnson, Asst. Exec. Dir.
New Jersey Board of Nursing
P.O. Box 45010
Newark, NJ 07101
Tel.: (201) 504-6430

Nancy L. Twigg, Exec. Dir.
New Mexico Board of Nursing
4206 Louisiana N.E., Suite A
Albuquerque, NM 87109
Tel.: (505) 841-8340

Milene A. Sower, Exec. Sec.
New York State Board of Nursing
The Cultural Center, Room 3023
Albany, NY 12230
Tel.: (518) 486-2967

Carol A. Osman, Exec. Dir.
North Carolina Board of
Nursing
P.O. Box 2129
Raleigh, NC 27602
Tel.: (919) 782-3211

Ida Rigley, Exec. Dir.
North Dakota Board of Nursing
919 S. 7th St., Suite 504
Bismarck, ND 58504-5881
Tel.: (701) 328-9777

Dorothy Fiorino, Exec. Dir.
Ohio Board of Nursing
77 S. High St., 17th Floor
Columbus, OH 43266-0316
Tel.: (614) 466-9800

Sulinda Moffett, Exec. Dir.
Oklahoma Board of Nursing
2915 N. Classen Blvd., Suite 524
Oklahoma City, OK 73106
Tel.: (405) 525-2076

Joan Bouchard, Exec. Dir.
Oregon State Board of Nursing
800 N.E. Oregon St., #25
Portland, OR 97232
Tel.: (503) 731-4745

Miriam H. Limo, Exec. Sec.
Pennsylvania State Board of
   Nursing
P.O. Box 2649
Harrisburg, PA 17105
Tel.: (717) 783-7142

Dr. Eusebio Diaz, Acting Dir.
Madeline Quilichini Paz, Dir.
Council on Higher Education of PR
P.O. Box 19900 F Juncos Sta.
San Juan, PR 00910-1900
Tel.: (787) 724-7100

Patricia Molloy, Dir.
Board of Nsg. Educ. and Nurse
   Registration
3 Capitol Hill
Providence, RI 02908-5097
Tel.: (401) 277-2827

Maggie Johnson, Interim Manager
State Board of Nursing for South
   Carolina
220 Executive Center Dr.,
   Suite 220
Columbia, SC 29210
Tel.: (803) 731-1648

Gloria Damgaard, Educ.
   Specialist
South Dakota Board of Nursing
3307 South Lincoln
Sioux Falls, SD 57105
Tel.: (605) 367-5940

Elizabeth J. Lund, RN,
   Exec. Dir.
Tennessee Board of Nursing
283 Plus Park Blvd.
Nashville, TN 37217
Tel.: (615) 532-5166

Katherine Thomas, Exec. Dir.
Texas Board of Nurse Examiners
333 Guadalupe, Box 140466
Austin, TX 78714
Tel.: (512) 305-7400

Laura Poe, Exec. Admin.
Utah State Board of Nursing
160 E. 300 South, Box 45805
Salt Lake City, UT 84145
Tel.: (801) 530-6628

Anita Ristau, Exec. Dir.
Vermont Board of Nursing,
   Licensing and Registration
   Divison
109 State St.
Montpelier, VT 05602
Tel.: (802) 828-2396

Winifred Garfield, Exec. Sec.
Virgin Islands Board of
   Nursing Licensure
P.O. Box 4247
Charolotte Amelie, VI 00803
Tel.: (809) 776-7397

Nancy Durrett, RN, Exec. Dir.
Virginia State Board of Nursing
6606 W. Broad St., 4th Floor
Richmond, VA 23230-1717
Tel.: (804) 662-9951

Patty Hayes, Exec. Dir.
Washington State Nursing Care
Quality Assurance Commission
1300 Quince Box 47864
Olympia, WA 98504-7864
Tel.: (360) 664-4208

Laura Rhodes, Exec. Sec.
Board of Examiners for Registered
  Nurses
101 Dee Dr.
Charleston, WV 25311-1620
Tel.: (304) 558-3596

Thomas Neumann, Admin. Off.
Wisconsin Dept. of Regulation &
  Licensing
P.O. Box 8935
Madison, WI 53708-8935
Tel.: (608) 267-2357

Toma Nisbet, Exec. Dir.
State of Wyoming Board of
  Nursing
2301 Central Ave., Barrett Bldg.
Cheyenne, WY 82002
Tel.: (307) 777-6127

Index

BEGINNING RN STUDY

LPN STUDY

BACCALAUREATE COMPLETION FOR RNs

ADVANCED CLINICAL STUDY FOR RNs

GRADUATE STUDY
(MASTER'S OR DOCTORAL)

DOCTORAL STUDY ONLY

SPECIAL AWARDS, POSTDOCTORAL STUDY, AND RESEARCH GRANTS

AID FOR MINORITY STUDENTS

NLN'S CONSTITUENT LEAGUES FOR NURSING

NURSING SPECIALTIES